A History of The London Clinic
A Celebration of 75 Years

A History of The London Clinic

A Celebration of 75 Years

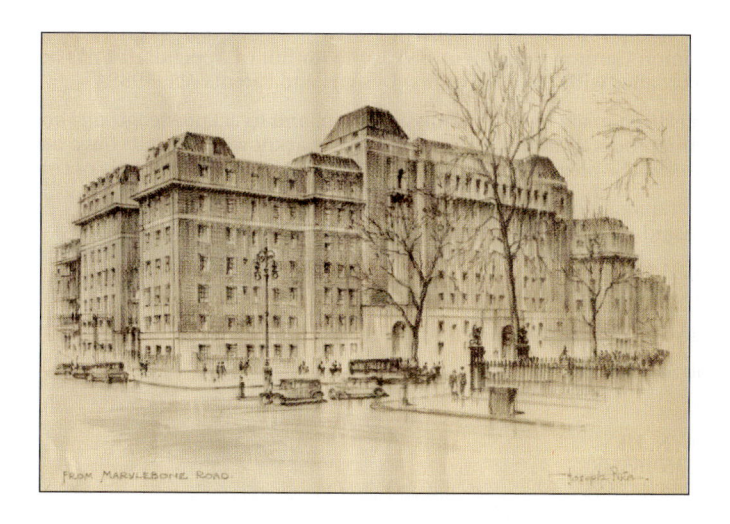

Harvey White

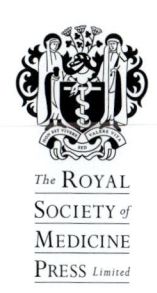

The ROYAL SOCIETY of MEDICINE PRESS Limited

the London clinic

© 2007 Royal Society of Medicine Press Ltd

Published by the Royal Society of Medicine Press Ltd
1 Wimpole Street, London W1G 0AE, UK
Tel: +44 (0)20 7290 2921
Fax: +44 (0)20 7290 2929
Email: publishing@rsm.ac.uk
Website: www.rsmpress.co.uk

Apart from any fair dealing for the purposes of research or private study, criticism or review, as permitted under the UK Copyright, Designs and Patents Act, 1988, no part of this publication may be reproduced, stored or transmitted, in any form or by any means, without the prior permission in writing of the publishers or in the case of reprographic reproduction in accordance with the terms of licences issued by the Copyright Licensing Agency in the UK, or in accordance with the terms of licences issued by the appropriate Reproduction Rights Organization outside the UK. Enquiries concerning reproduction outside the terms stated here should be sent to the publishers at the UK address printed on this page.

The right of Harvey White to be identified as author of this work has been asserted by him in accordance with the Copyrights, Designs and Patents Act, 1988.

The right of Simon Gannon to be identified as the Author of Appendix 14 has been asserted by him in accordance with the Copyrights, Designs and Patents Act, 1988.

Every effort has been made to seek permission from, and to acknowledge, all those whose work has been reproduced in this publication. If any acknowledgements have been overlooked, we will be pleased to include these in any subsequent editions of this publication.

British Library Cataloguing in Publication Data
A catalogue record for this book is available from the British Library

ISBN 978-1-85315-679-3 (pbk)
ISBN 978-1-85315-712-7 (hbk)

Distribution in Europe and Rest of World:

Marston Book Services Ltd
PO Box 269
Abingdon
Oxon OX14 4YN, UK
Tel: +44 (0)1235 465500
Fax: +44 (0)1235 465555
Email: direct.order@marston.co.uk

Distribution in the USA and Canada:

Royal Society of Medicine Press Ltd
c/o BookMasters Inc
30 Amberwood Parkway
Ashland, OH 44805, USA
Tel: +1 800 247 6553/+1 800 266 5564
Fax: +1 419 281 6883
Email: order@bookmasters.com

Distribution in Australia and New Zealand:

Elsevier Australia
30–52 Smidmore Street
Marrickville NSW 2204, Australia
Tel: +61 2 9517 8999
Fax: +61 2 9517 2249
Email: service@elsevier.com.au

Typeset by Phoenix Photosetting, Chatham, Kent
Printed by Alfabase, The Netherlands

Contents

	Foreword	vii
	Harvey White	ix
	Preface	xi
	Acknowledgements	xv
1	Historical introduction	1
2	Beginnings	11
3	Buildings	17
4	Top brass and general headquarters – the godlike kings of old	25
5	Ranfurly and Ramsden years	31
6	The third way	41
7	Patients	51
8	The good, the bad and the ugly	55
9	Nursing	61
10	Physiotherapy, phlebotomists and interpreters	71
11	Catering	73
12	Trace elements – clinical essentials	79
13	The front line – 149 Harley Street	83
14	The heroes of old	91
15	Spinning a yarn	93
16	Theatres	99
17	Radiology, radiotherapy and imaging	109
18	Endoscopy	113
19	Pathology and pharmacy	117

20	Making it happen – house governors and chief executive	123
21	Information technology	125
22	Lest we forget and *The London Clinic Medical Journal*	127
23	Veterans and Christmas	133
24	We have lift off	137

Appendices 143

1	Acknowledgements listing	145
2	Clinic mission and philosophy	147
3	Chairmen, house governors, chief executive and matrons	149
4	Governors and trustees, operations board and executive board	151
5	Medical advisory committee, chairmen of the medical advisory committee and specialty user groups, 2007	153
6	Charitable status	155
7	The London Clinic: committee structure	159
8	The London Clinic: organizational charts	161
9	Celebrity openings of departments	165
10	*The London Clinic Medical Journal* listings of clinical articles	171
11	*The London Clinic Medical Journal* listings of non-clinical articles	179
12	Obituary of Sir Aynsley Bridgland	181
13	Explosive ordnance threat assessment of The London Clinic Cancer Centre	185
14	An archaeological evaluation report	245
15	The effect of Prime Minister Anthony Eden's illness on his decision-making during the Suez crisis	271
	Index	273

Foreword

I am immensely proud to be a Trustee of The London Clinic and so it gives me great pleasure to write the Foreword to this book which reflects 75 years of service and dedication on the part of those who have worked and continue to work at The London Clinic.

It has been written by Harvey White, a truly remarkable man, the ideal author for a fascinating book covering much more than the bare bones about the history of the Clinic. Formerly a practising surgeon at The London Clinic for over thirty years, Harvey White has already written many books on medical history: here however he has given his wonderful sense of humour full rein and the book contains many amusing anecdotes, interesting historical facts and journeys into the byways of poetry and prose from many unusual sources.

It is 75 years since the late Queen Elizabeth, the Queen Mother, officially opened The London Clinic in 1932. Since then, particularly in recent years, it has become one of the leading independent hospitals not only in this country but throughout the world.

Its specialities, which include Cancer treatments, Hepatology, Neurosciences, Orthopaedics/Spinal, Endocrinology/Diabetes, Gastroenterology, Gastrointestinal/Colorectal, Gynaecology, Ophthalmology, Oral/Maxillofacial, E.N.T., Plastic/Aesthetic, Thoracic and Vascular are all at the cutting edge of technology. The practitioners who take their patients to the Clinic are universally respected as consultants of great knowledge and skill.

The London Clinic has a reputation which is second to none for the quality of its nursing care. This has been developed over the 75 years of its history: patients with acute and difficult illnesses come from all over the world to receive treatment there. In this book Harvey White has unmasked his colleagues and shown us what lies behind the screens.

The Duchess of Devonshire DL

CLARENCE HOUSE
S.W.1

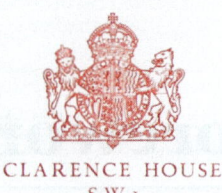

Just sixty years ago it was my pleasure to perform the opening of the London Clinic. Since that far off February day in 1932 the Clinic has gone from strength to strength, in peace and war, providing medical skill, brilliant surgery and devoted nursing to patients of every age and background.

May its splendid amenities continue to be of benefit to mankind in the years ahead. To all those who serve at the Clinic - to the doctors, surgeons and members of the nursing and ancillary staff I offer my greetings and best wishes in this Jubilee Year.

ELIZABETH R
Queen Mother

February 1992

Harvey White

Harvey White was a consultant surgeon at the Royal Marsden Hospital when most of his private work was undertaken at The London Clinic from his rooms in 95 Harley Street. After retiring from the NHS, he spent more than 15 years in rooms at 149 Harley Street (below) and served on numerous Clinic committees. Apart from a wide range of clinical publications, he has written extensively on the history of medicine and surgery.

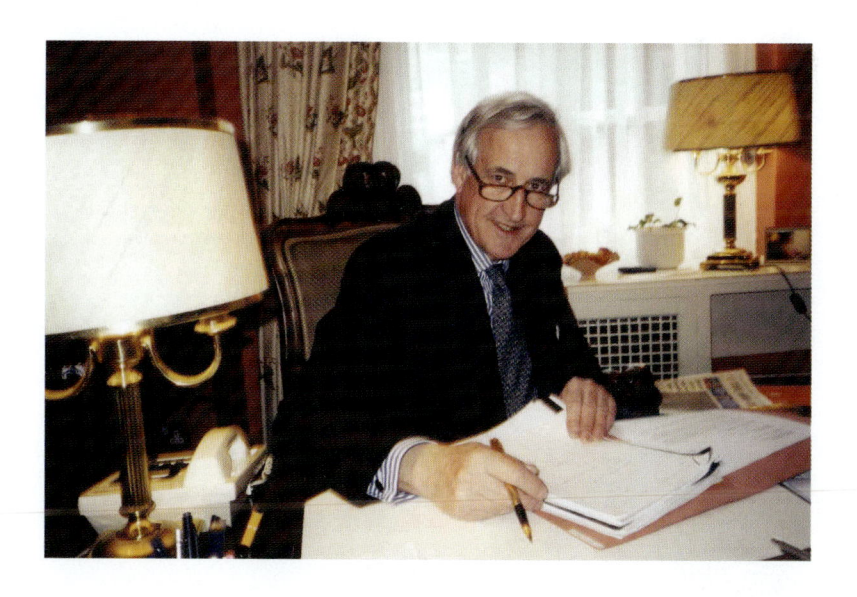

Preface

Some might think it is rather presumptuous of me to agree to write a history of The London Clinic. The undertaking is somewhat daunting and it was not until I came to write this preface that my thoughts were crystallized as to what sort of a book I should write. At first I thought a professional historian should undertake the task – a dedicated work of scholarship, perhaps. On mulling this over I felt such an archive was not required – and it would not find a wide readership. I then thought I could edit a book with sections written by those in the various departments which make up the Clinic. The chairman, in his wisdom, did not agree, and I therefore undertook the task.

I took a decision to write an account of the Clinic that drew on the personal memories of patients, nursing staff, specialists and administrators. Many of these might seem better placed to do justice to the task that I am attempting, but I cannot betray the trust that has been placed in me. The important thing is that it should be recorded while those who have been privileged to spend part of their working life in the Clinic are still able to contribute their memories – especially as many records are missing and probably permanently lost. Included among these are early minute books and even records of the appointment of matrons.

I feel a responsibility to capture the character and ethos of the place, as I owe a debt of gratitude to have been able to make it my clinical home after leaving the NHS. It has been a happy and fulfilling time. I hope to preserve and record the past so that those in a changing world can understand how the ethos and traditions of the place have become enshrined in the folklore and reality of a unique institution.

This is, therefore, not to be a dull history – not that any history is or ever should be dull. History is, of course, a dialogue with the past that we ignore at our peril. From it we understand our beginnings and the way we conduct our lives; we also determine where we are heading or, to be more precise, where the next generation are going and where they will take the Clinic. I hope to capture the character of the place, the excellence that underlies the endeavours of all the staff and the personalities of some of those who have made it what it is. It is not just a nursing home and hospital; it is an institution that in many ways is part of our national heritage.

The Clinic has meant so many different things to so many that it will be difficult to place it in context for all. Patients become attached to the place and often have a fierce loyalty and a love of the staff who have cared for them. The morale and dedication of the nursing staff is relied on by the medical specialists. They themselves regard it as a haven of excellence from the often troubled world of the NHS in which they spend much of their time. In effect, it is the best medical club in Europe.

All of this must be told and recorded before it is lost. The changes taking place in the delivery of healthcare are rapid and far reaching. Hopefully, the Clinic will be able to graft these onto the tradition of the institution without losing all those aspects that we love and feel to be important. It is an exceptional institution with its own character and legends, which I hope will come to light in the following pages and will be interesting and make good reading for patients and staff alike. In addition to the many sources and memories of those connected with the Clinic, I have drawn heavily on the history written by Willi Frischauer in 1967. I make full acknowledgment of this and much of the material and stories from that book will now have a welcome renaissance. Some repetition between the sections allows each to stand alone more comfortably for those with only enough energy or interest to dip into the book before succumbing to Morpheus.

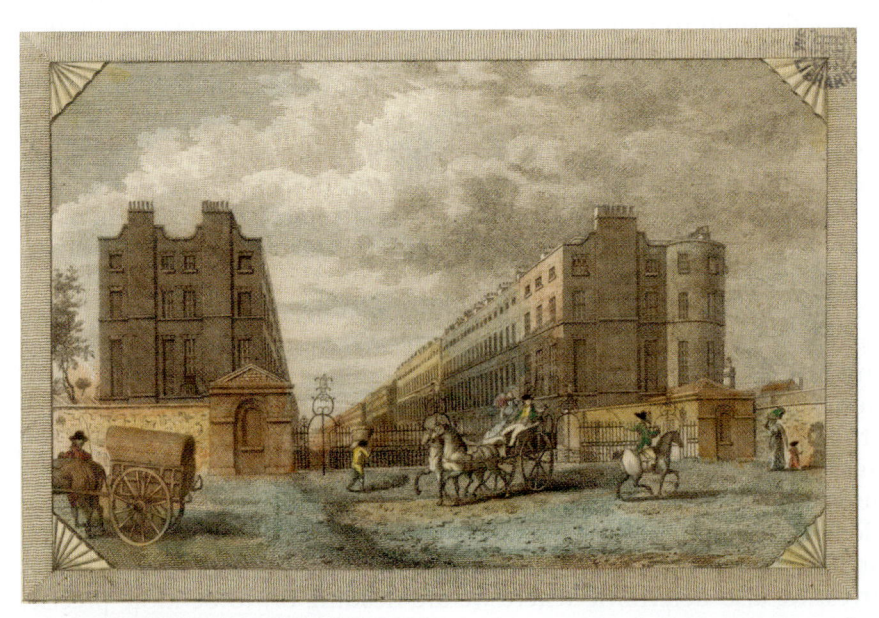

Devonshire Place and Wimpole Street from the New Road, St Mary Le Bone, September 1793. Reproduced with kind permission from the City of Westminster Archives Centre.

If I fail in my task I will not do justice to the Clinic or to the patients and staff who have made it what it is.

Let it be a celebration of seventy five years!

In salutem praesentium in memoriam absentium

Acknowledgements

I am grateful for many verbal and written contributions. Most of these are listed in Appendix 1, and I hope that anyone unwittingly omitted will be forgiving. I have received much encouragement, support and information not only from the chairman and chief executive and their predecessors but also the directors and their directorates. The universal enthusiasm and help that has been willingly given in support of this little project has been pleasantly reassuring.

In the preface, I have already made reference to the book about the Clinic by Willi Frischauer (1967),[1] from which many of the patient anecdotes have been drawn.

This book would probably not have reached completion – certainly not in its present form – were it not for Kathy Perkins. Her research and enthusiasm has been essential and compelling both in sourcing old documents and creating a picture archive. She has tolerated my varied and old-fashioned methods of working and blended them with her electronic literacy, for which I have great admiration. In addition to my own debt, the Clinic should be grateful that she has laid the foundations for a permanent archive.

Sheila Hartley has been a painstaking and willing transcriber of tapes and medical handwriting. Her loyalty and efficiency continued despite her husband's terminal illness, and I pay tribute to and thank her.

The RSM Press, led by my friend Peter Richardson, has been very friendly, supportive and efficient. I have relied heavily on this not only now but for the eight years during which I was their chairman. The Project Editor, Hannah Wessely, has steered the book through editing and production most efficiently, enabling the publication deadline to be met in time for the 75th anniversary celebrations. I am also grateful to Gabi Mills for coming out of maternal retirement to proof-read another book of mine.

Dr D Geraint James kindly read the manuscript, and his corrections and suggestions have been invaluable.

I thank my family and friends who have been characteristically understanding during my preoccupation with this project!

Reference
1. Frischauer W. *The Clinic*. London: Leslie Frewin Publishers, 1967.

1

Historical introduction

London grew up along the banks of the Thames. There were fortifications such as the Tower of London and Castle Baynard. Trade flourished in markets like Billingsgate, adjacent to the docks and the quays. Along the banks were a number of developments, including royal palaces such as Greenwich and Westminster. Residential property was built around these palaces and flourishing communities developed to support the court. Hospitals were founded on the north and south banks of the Thames – St Bartholomew's, Guys and Thomas's being the oldest. Doctors lived close to these hospitals and also in proximity to the royal palaces. One such was Robert Balthrop, whose parents lived by Greenwich Palace. He eventually lived within the hospital precinct of St Bartholomew and became sergeant surgeon to Elizabeth I.

As the city grew, farms and communities developed along the banks of rivers like the Fleet and Tyburn, which flowed along what is now Tachbrook Street in Pimlico and into the Thames. Radial roads ran to the north and south, eventually becoming joined by orbital roads. One of these to the north was New Road, which ran to the east from the church of St Mary-at-the-Bourne. This eventually became Maribone (or Marylebone) Road. This marked the boundary between a large residential development and the deer park of Maribone (now Regent's Park), which was created by Henry VIII (1509–47). The dissolution of the monasteries (1536–40) changed the history of Marylebone, which nestled on the edge of the royal hunting ground. Having appropriated the revenue of Tyburn (30 shillings a year), the king then acquired the whole manor of Tyburn and enparked it. Some circumstantial evidence suggests that the king traced out the boundary himself – to the detriment of the local landowners. In 1539, one, Thomas Hobson, was offered several houses near Southampton in exchange, including the Manor of Colbury, where, by the strangest coincidence, I spent some of my childhood. The King granted the Manor of Tyburn to Sir Anthony Denny, a privy counsellor and keeper of Westminster Palace. A ring mound was created around the park to retain the deer and exclude poachers. This is the origin of the outer circle.

The residential area associated with the Manor of Tyburn, which had been procured by the king three years before his death, was sold to George Cavendish (1500–61), who was in constant attendance on Cardinal Wolsey and became his usher in 1526. He ultimately became Wolsey's biographer. George Cavendish died around 1561, and his younger brother William (1505–57) received grants of land from Henry VIII in return for securing the property of the monasteries at the dissolution (1536–40). Henry VIII knighted him on 25 April 1546. He married Elizabeth, known as 'Bess of Hardwicke', who previously had been married to Robert Barlow. After the purchase of the Chatsworth estate in 1549, she started the development of the great house in 1552. In all, she had four husbands. After Robert Barlow and Sir William Cavendish, she married Sir William St Loe and ultimately in 1568 George Talbot, the sixth Earl of Shrewsbury. She inherited estates from all four of her husbands and had an estimated annual income of £60,000 a year in the late 1880s (the equivalent today would be nearly £8m).

William, the second son of Sir William Cavendish and Bess of Hardwicke, was a courtier to James I and a member of parliament for Liverpool (1586) and Newport, Cornwall (1589). He became the first Earl of Devonshire in 1618, just six years before his death. His sister married Gilbert Talbot, the seventh Earl of Shrewsbury. The names, the lives and the lands of the Cavendish and Talbot families therefore became inextricably mixed, and the Devonshire name lives on in the area, as does the Shrewsbury Association, which is perpetuated in Welbeck Street, as Welbeck Abbey was their country seat. The present Duchess of Devonshire is a governor of The London Clinic.

Crown ownership of the park continued until 1645, when Charles I was short of funds and pledged it to Sir George Strode and John Wandesford. The manor house of Tyburn was leased to Edward Forsett by Elizabeth I (1558–1603). James I (1603–25) ultimately sold it to Forsett in 1611 for £8,291.3.4p.

After the Treaty of Utrecht in 1713, which concluded the great European war of the Spanish succession, England obtained, among other territories, possession of Newfoundland, Nova Scotia and Gibraltar. The treaty with France at this time recognized the protestant succession in England. Peace brought stability and economic confidence and with it new life to the London property market. Investment rates fell and feverish building took place between 1716 and 1718.

London continued to grow and was developed by the great families. Marriage bonds at that time were effectively property bonds. Great estates were created as a result of marriages such as those between the second Earl of Cadogan and Elizabeth Sloane in 1717 and Sir Thomas Grosvenor and the heiress Mary Davis (a girl of 12 years) in 1677.

Lady Margaret Cavendish, daughter and co-heiress of the Duke of

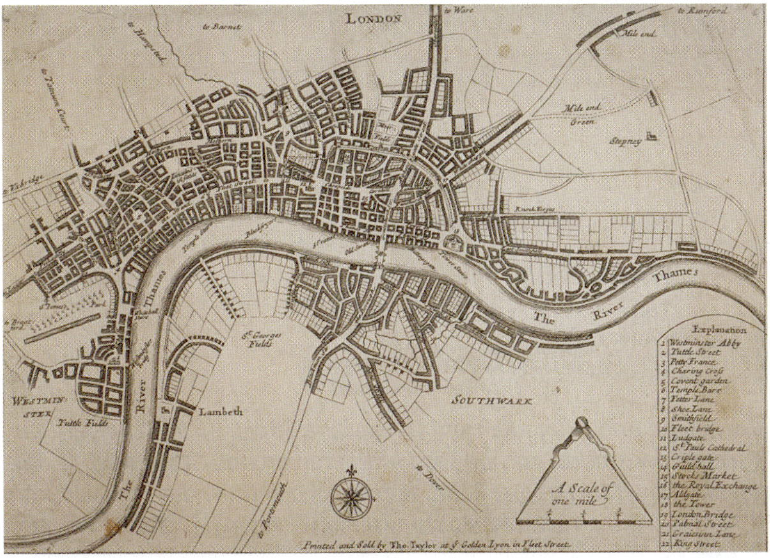

Historical introduction

Figure 1.1 *Map of London, 1716, showing the City, Westminster, Lambeth and Southwark. Reproduced with kind permission from Guildhall Library, City of London.*

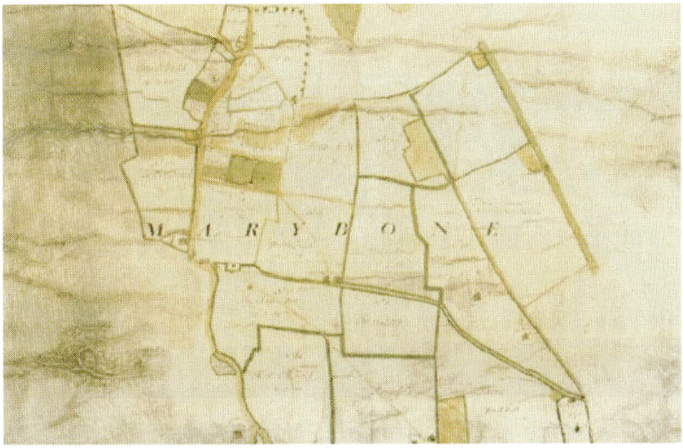

Figure 1.2 *Map of Marylebone, 1708, by Henry Pratt, showing that the area was mainly farmland at that time. Reproduced with kind permission from the Howard de Walden Estate.*

Newcastle, became the second wife of John Holles, Earl of Clare. He was a friend and political ally of Robert Harley, son of Sir Edward Harley. Harley was high sheriff of Herefordshire and a prominent Tory who became chancellor of the exchequer, initiating a scheme for funding the national debt through the South Sea Company. He had also been responsible for obtaining the creation of 12 new peers to carry the Treaty of Utrecht in 1713.

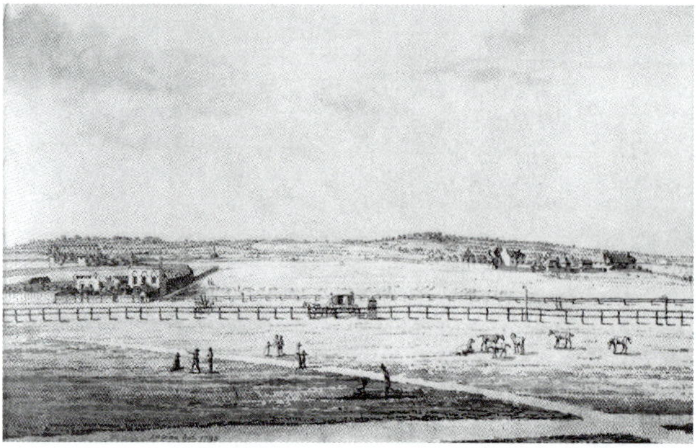

Figure 1.3 *Hampstead and Highgate from Devonshire Street, 1793. Dupper Field, where Park Crescent now stands, can be seen in the foreground. The coach is driving along New Road, now Marylebone Road. Reproduced with kind permission from the British Museum. © British Library Board. All rights reserved. Shelfmark Add. 15542 Folio N. 136.*

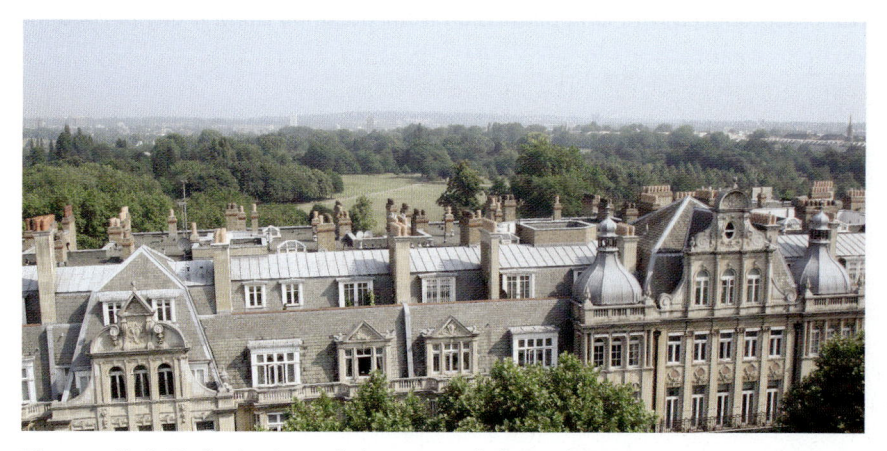

Figure 1.4 *Today's view of the same skyline, showing Hampstead Heath in the sky-line.*

The trading and manipulation of honours is not new, and Harley himself had been created Earl of Oxford and Mortimer in 1711. His country seat was Wimpole in Cambridgeshire, and he also owned an estate at Wigmore. Both names are perpetuated as streets in the area. Edward Harley's daughter, Margaret Cavendish-Holles-Harley, married William Bentink, the second Duke of Portland, in 1734. This completed the somewhat incestuous association of great families that dictated and defined the map from Cavendish Square to Marylebone Road and became known as the Portland Estate.

Historical introduction

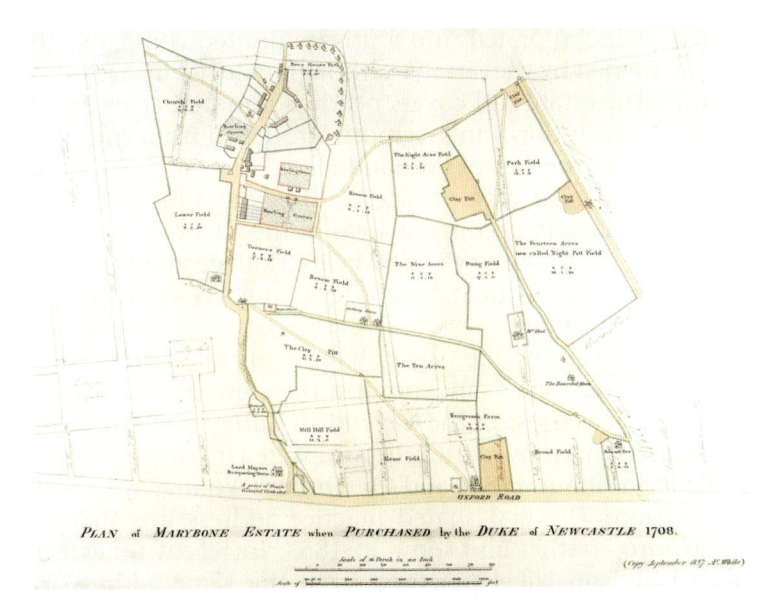

Figure 1.5 Henry Pratt's plan of the Marylebone Estate when purchased by the Duke of Newcastle, 1708. It includes a reference to Dove House Park (site of the new cancer centre). Reproduced with kind permission from the Crace Collection, British Library. © British Library Board. All rights reserved. port. XV1.18.

The area gradually became associated with excellence in private medicine for the benefit of the well-to-do. The development at Cavendish Square initially faltered when investors withdrew their money after the South Sea crash of 1720. It was not completed until some 50 years after the original plans were made.

Harley Street was able to develop when the reservoir north of Cavendish Square was dismantled. The street was first rated in 1753 and was a smart residential area. The artist JMW Turner moved into number 64 in 1804 and the Duchess of Wellington to number 11 in 1809. Queen's College, the first school for the higher education of women, occupied numbers 43–49 from 1848 onwards, and the Florence Nightingale Hospital moved from Lisson Grove to 1 Harley Street in 1853. Gladstone moved into 73 Harley Street in 1876, just three years before the death of the fifth Duke of Portland, who was childless. The estate then passed jointly to his three sisters. Two of the sisters (Charlotte and Harriet) died, leaving the estate as the sole inheritance of Lucy, the widow of the sixth Lord Howard de Walden, who had died in 1868. The estate, formerly known as the Portland Estate, then became the Howard de Walden Estate in 1879 and has remained in the ownership of the Howard de Walden family since then. The barony recently passed to Lady Howard de Walden, the eldest daughter of the late ninth Lord Howard.

In 1918, the estate was incorporated into a private limited company, all the shares of which are owned by the family. Although reduced in size from the nineteenth century, the estate still covers nearly a hundred acres, from Marylebone Road in the north down to Wigmore Street and from the west of Marylebone High Street to the east of Portland Place.

Just as courtiers had lived near royal palaces in previous times, doctors lived near their hospitals – largely occupying areas in the City and Bloomsbury in order to be near St Bartholomew's, University College and the Middlesex Hospitals. Mayfair was favoured by those at the Westminster, St Thomas's and St George's Hospitals.

As time went on and travel became easier, it was possible and indeed more pleasant to live further afield and occupy the new developments north of Oxford Street, such as those of the Cavendish Harley Estate. Two of the first doctors known to have moved into the area were Dr James Latham, who took up residence in about 1880, and Dr Thomas Young, who was interested in colour vision. The first shared practice address was that of Edward and Henry Monro – father and son – in 1853. In recent times, Sir Ralph Southward and his son Nigel practised from the same address in Devonshire Place. Inevitably, the quacks – represented, among others, by John Long – were opportunists and followed close on the heels of early respectable physicians.

Professional advertising was not allowed, but a discreet brass plate was acceptable, and specialists used their dining rooms as waiting rooms. This was the thin end of the wedge, and market forces were destined to drive the lettings. By 1904, there were 200 licence plates, and, by 1932, when The London Clinic was opened, some 900. No wonder there was a need for a nursing home in the area. Most teaching hospitals had some private beds – but not St Bartholomew's, where it was prevented by the Royal Charter when the hospital was refounded by Henry VIII after the dissolution of the monasteries. These private facilities, however, were not sufficient. The proximity of the medical institutions, such as the Royal Society of Medicine and Medical Society of London, further defined the medical character of the area.

Even if not naturally gregarious, doctors tend to become so during their training and apprenticeship. This carries on during their working lives, and one benefit of being in close proximity is the opportunity to obtain second opinions from colleagues. There is nothing like trust and cooperation to underpin market forces, and it was not long before the area had an established national and international reputation for medical excellence.

The medical journal *The Lancet* was not slow to comment on the tendency of the wealthy hypochondriacs to prefer an address to a degree, however, but for all that there was no shortage of good doctors or good opinions. Those who paid liked to relate to their medical advisers and feel comfortable in the advice that was being meted out. They undoubtedly sought the advice of those who effectively supported their own views about what was good for them. WH Auden succinctly captures this relationship:

Historical introduction

> '*Give me a doctor partridge plump*
> *Short in the leg and broad in the rump*
> *An endomorph with gentle hands*
> *Who'll never make absurd demands*
> *That I abandon all my vices*
> *Nor pull a long face in a crisis*
> *But with a twinkle in his eye*
> *Will tell me that I have to die*'

It was not really as bad as the detractors would suggest. Michèle Stokes[1] in her study of the development of Harley Street as a centre of medical excellence has analysed the published work, editing of journals and public lectures undertaken by those who put up their plates in the Street. On each count, they outshone other practising doctors in London, and 75% held senior staff positions against 10% of a matched group practising in the rest of London. In 1914, 39% were physicians and 37% surgeons, with more than 50% being fellows of their respective royal colleges compared with 1% elsewhere in London.

The names of the great in the profession were to be seen up and down the Street on brass plates. Some of the illustrious are still recorded on heritage plaques – examples are Sir Frederick Treeves, who removed the appendix of Edward VII before the delayed coronation, and Sir Ronald Ross, who helped to identify and resolve some of the mosquito-related health problems that were experienced by members of the British army in the far flung corners of the empire. Sir Jonathan Hutchinson, the surgeon who described an anomaly of the pupils of the eyes, lived on the north side of Cavendish Square.

Specialists used to own or rent a house in which their families lived and they conducted their private practice. This still happened in the 1960s, and I can remember parties in 134 Harley Street, which was inhabited solely by Sir Ronald Bodley Scott. Two of the last of my colleagues to live in this exalted way were the oncologist Ronald Raven, who occupied number 29 until his death in 1991, and another surgeon, Lionel Gracey. The great men (and there really were very few women then, even after the pioneering era of Elizabeth Garrett Anderson) used to travel in chauffeur-driven cars from the mews at the back of their houses to the hospitals, where, before the advent of the NHS in 1948, they would have practised in a voluntary capacity.

Few laboratories were required in those days and but little diagnostic equipment. Portable electrocardiograms and facilities for simple x-rays sufficed. As expectations developed, simple procedures were undertaken in consulting rooms. One of the more adventurous in this respect was by the radiologist from St Bartholomew's Hospital, Dr MS Finzi. He occupied one of the basements just down from 149 Harley Street, using it for electrical and radium treatment.

Those who could afford the rents gradually diminished, and the pressures for more licences grew. Something of a cartel was in place, operated by the

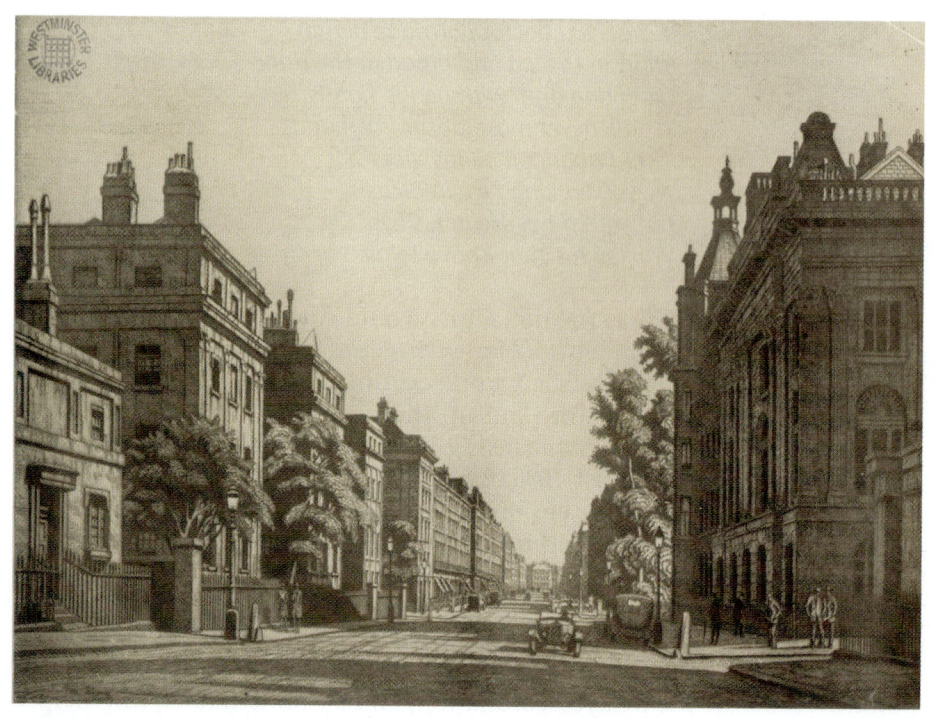

Figure 1.6 Harley Street 1928, known as 'The Road of Life and Death'. Original etching by Ian Strang. Reproduced with kind permission from the City of Westminster Archives Centre.

ground landlords – chiefly the Howard de Walden Estate and the Crown Estates. Single occupancy was becoming unusual, basements and attics were turned into apartments with the disappearance of servants and the main rooms of the house became consulting suites for visiting specialists – either for full-time renting or as a sessional half day. Pressure grew for more licences, but this was initially resisted for fear that it would debase the undoubted prestige associated with 'putting up a plate in Harley Street'. This was self-defeating, as only the exceptional specialists who could command extremely high fees and those who exploited the misfortune of the sick were able to afford the overheads.

Hilaire Belloc captures the social and professional cultures in two of his cautionary tales:

> 'Physicians of the utmost fame
> Were called at once but when they came
> They answered as they took their fees
> There is no cure for this disease.'

Historical introduction

> 'To bed! To bed and do not speak
> A single word till Wednesday week
> When I will come and set you free
> (If you are cured) and take my fee!'[2]

The Victorian drawing room culture continued to be the expected environment in which consultations were undertaken, and a minimum of clinical furniture and white coats were to be found amidst a maximum of awe, affability and availability. Of course, there had to be a show of enough opulence and self-confidence to underpin the fees and confirm the value of the professional opinion that was given without even a thought of discussing the fees first (that would have smacked of trade).

The professional life was secure, ordered and affluent. The elegant properties in the area were ideal and staff both affordable and plentiful. The trust of patients was infinite, and respect meant that opinions seldom were questioned. Professional charity was dispensed not only within the great hospitals around London but also on occasion to the less fortunate who found their way to 'the Street' seeking second opinions for life-threatening situations. Hand-in-hand with the social upheaval after the First World War, medicine was becoming more objective and diagnosis more dependent on science and measurement. The support of pathology departments became inseparable from the Victorian drawing room culture. The need for inpatient facilities for nursing care, physiotherapy and invasive procedures grew. In addition, early statistics showed that in certain cases – including home deliveries – it was statistically safer to be in a nursing home.

Visionary thinking and an entrepreneurial spirit led to the consulting room culture in Harley Street being supplemented by The London Clinic. This colossus developed astride the north end of Devonshire Place and Harley Street – like a mother ship to a flotilla of submarines, able to supply all the requirements not available to those spearheading the attack on disease in their consulting rooms, whether diagnostic or therapeutic.

The elegant houses with Georgian proportions – some decorated with fine and rare examples of Coade stone finials – were now dwarfed by the Clinic's building, making a grand statement and radiating confidence. It could well be referred to as the terracotta dowager of Harley Street, in the way that John Betjeman was later to describe Harrods. The telegraphic address of Harrods used to be 'Everything, London'. The Clinic set out to provide a similar comprehensive service in the field of medicine. How did it all happen? What were the trials and tribulations of the project both before it was built and after the doors were opened in 1932. How did it come to be the most important private clinic in the country and one that was envied around the world? The story must be recorded and the atmosphere and ethos captured before they are lost in the cauldron of change that is overtaking our once-secure professional world. Let us remember those wise words of Winston Churchill, 'The longer you look back, the further you look forward.'

References
1. Michèle Stokes. A Measure of the Elite: A history of medical practitioners in Harley Street, 1845–1914 [dissertation]. London: University College London, 2004.
2. Hilaire Belloc text is reproduced by permission of PFD (www.pfd.co.uk) on behalf of the Estate of Hilaire Belloc. © The Estate of Hilaire Belloc, 1896.

2
Beginnings

London has always embraced extremes, catering for the richest and dispensing charity to the poorest but having comparative disregard for the middle classes and those who underpin the lives of the wealthy. Medicine was no exception, with the great hospitals for the poor and private nurses or nursing homes for the well-to-do. The medical needs of those from the services, the clergy and the professional classes had been rather neglected within the capital – apart from some of the hospitals dedicated to specific diseases such as the Brompton Chest Hospital and the Royal Marsden Cancer Hospital. Outside London, various hospitals such as Haslar and Botley were dedicated to the services. Some, such as the Royal Sea Bathing at Margate and the Hospital for Rheumatic Diseases in Bath, had specialist interests. In due course, hospitals in London were also founded for the services (Millbank, Woolwich and King Edward VII, which started as a nursing home for army officers in Grosvenor Crescent). There were also hospitals for the clergy, freemasons, members of the trade unions and other groups, all of which had some charitable aspects.

The pressure on beds and finances initially were of little importance at The London Clinic. Patients were admitted a night or two before their operation and were given ample time to regain their strength and confidence before returning home. It was not unusual for a husband to be admitted when his wife was awaiting delivery in the obstetric department, in which beds (as in the rest of the Clinic) could be pre-booked. Such luxuries had to be abandoned in the face of a changing world of financial pressures, medical insurance and the advent of day surgery.

In order to be a patient at the Clinic, it was necessary to be under the care of a doctor on the British Medical Register who himself had admitting rights – this applied both to specialists and general practitioners. These had to be approved by a small house committee, which included some of the prominent specialists themselves. They inevitably became powerful in regulating and protecting their own oligarchy. This, of course, was not unknown in the medical profession elsewhere in the country!

Before 1932, there had been a number of private nursing homes in London – Almina Carnarvon's Alfred House in Portland Place was largely restricted to the nobility. Mrs Miles, widow of Ernest Miles (the surgeon from the Royal Marsden Hospital who undertook the first abdominoperineal dissection), ran the nursing home in Fitzroy Square. There was even a nursing home (run by a widowed anaesthetist and Terrence Millin) at 31 Queensgate, where surgery was undertaken. It was here that retropubic prostatectomy was first perfected. One other nursing home – that in Vincent Square – undertook treatment with vestigial deep x-ray apparatus. In the vicinity of Harley Street, there was a nursing home run by Elizabeth Fulcher and one by Miss Cuncanson on the present site of King Edward VII's Hospital in Beaumont Street.

The London Clinic was the first institution in Britain for private patients to cater for all aspects of a modern hospital, supplying not only modern equipment but also a wide variety of services. It had a certain intimacy, privacy and friendliness that one would normally expect at home or in a small private nursing home. It held a standard Howard de Walden lease for a private dwelling house coupled with a separate licence to use the premises for the 'business of a Clinic and nursing home, proprietors and leasors of consulting rooms.' Fifty licences for consulting rooms were issued initially. This lease shows that from the outset it was the intention to provide both state-of-the-art clinical care and the intimacy and privacy of a small nursing home. The fees were seven guineas a week (inclusive as far as possible). Inside the complex, 36 physicians and surgeons had consulting rooms and two resident medical officers provided continuity of care. Most of the 214 rooms had adjoining bathrooms. The rooms were served by 200 nurses and 70 maids. The construction and equipment for the hospital was budgeted to cost £400,000 (equivalent to £9m today), but this was exceeded by some £50,000 (more than £1m today).

The title of the main premises started with a lease that was to run from 11 October 1929 for 95 years and nine months. The foundation stone was laid by the Duchess of Atholl on 29 November 1929. The annual rent of the site at that time was £2,075.

The Duchess of York, accompanied by the Duke of York (later King George VI), performed the opening on 18 February (Figures 2.1, 2.2 and 2.3). The previous Saturday afternoon the King (George V) and Queen Mary had visited the Clinic to meet the chairman and matron and inspect the porters. By this time, some patients were already installed (before the official opening). One of the nurses (Nurse Black) was a patient herself, and the King and Queen visited her as she had nursed the King during an illness four years previously. Dignitaries at the ceremony included the first Chairman of the Clinic (the Eighth Duke of Atholl), Lord Dawson of Penn (Figure 15.1) and Lord Moynihan (Figure 2.4) (physician and surgeon,

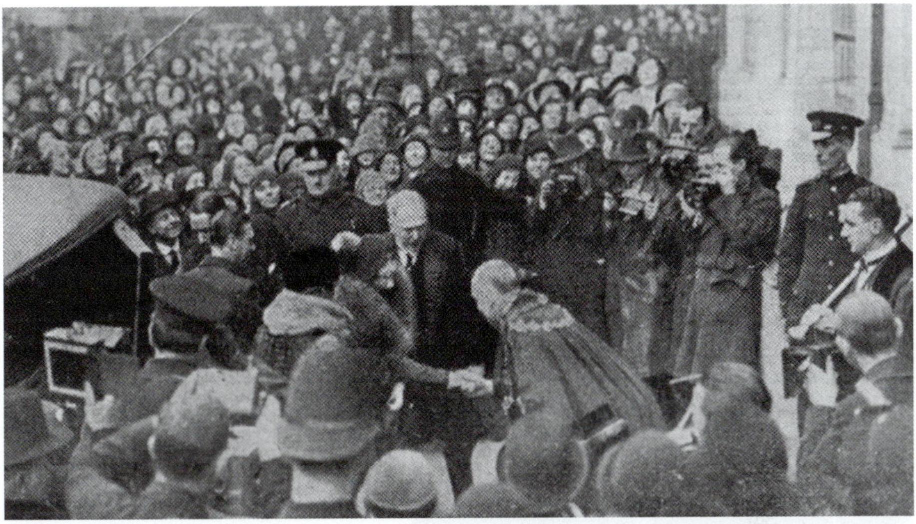

Beginnings 13

Figure 2.1 HRH The Duchess of York, accompanied by HRH The Duke of York, being welcomed on arrival at the Clinic.

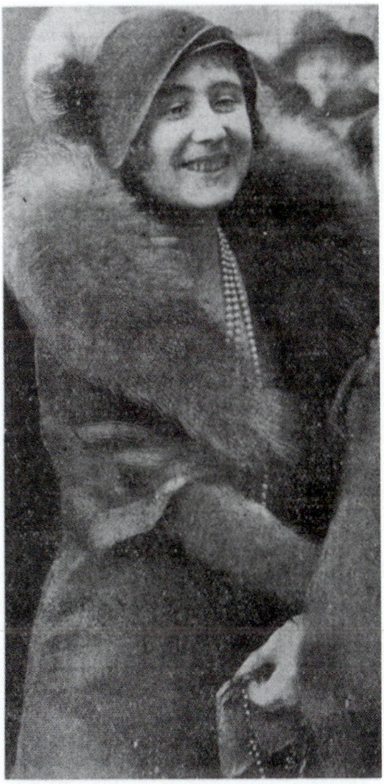

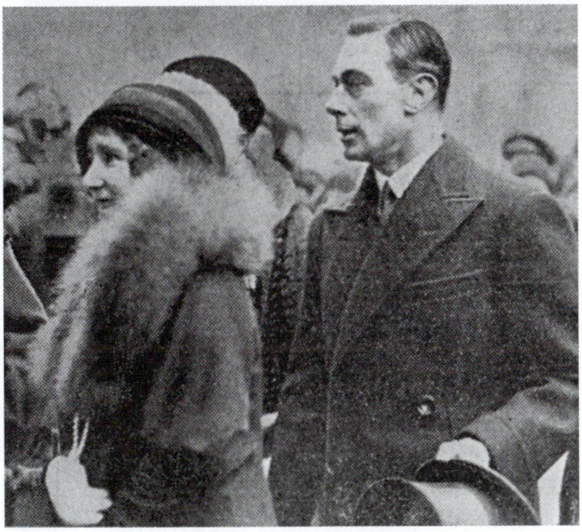

Figure 2.3 HRH The Duchess of York accompanied by HRH The Duke of York.

Figure 2.2 HRH The Duchess of York.

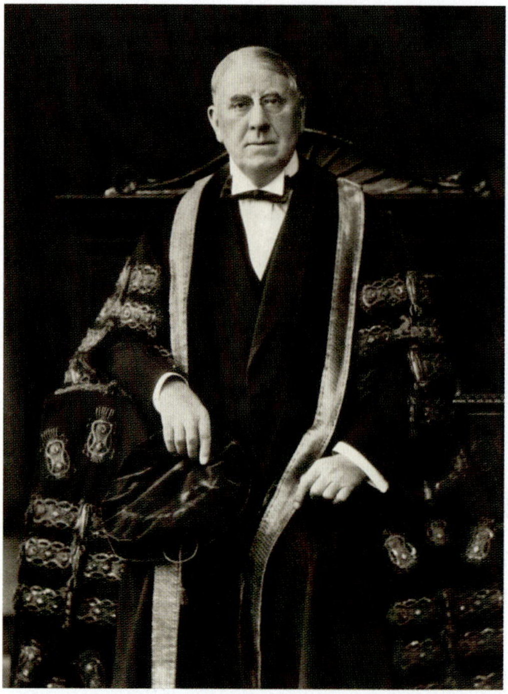

Figure 2.4 *Lord Moynihan. Reproduced with kind permission from the RSM Library.*

respectively), the house governor, Ernest William Morris (later Sir Ernest) and the matron, Miss Hebdon.

On the very day that the Clinic was opened by the Duchess, the independence of Manchuria was declared at a somewhat less glamorous ceremony. The same year, also, Ibn Saud declared Saudi Arabia to be a kingdom. The Clinic and that country have, as it were, grown hand-in-hand ever since.

The first 50 patients were admitted to the fifth floor (Figure 2.5), and the very first patient was Miss Margaret Balmer of Sheerwater Cottage, West Byfleet. Her shoulder required manipulation by the eminent orthopaedic surgeon – Rowley Bristow, of 102 Harley Street. In later years, a hospital named after him was opened in West Byfleet, which was his country retreat and close to where the first patient lived.

Other distinguished consultants who used the Clinic at the beginning were gynaecologists Victor Bonney and Sir Lenthal Cheatle and general surgeons Lord Moynihan of Leeds and Mr Lockhart Mummery (whose son Sir Lyn Lockhart Mummery was, in his time, also a consultant at the Clinic). Sir Harold Gillies had rooms on the ground floor of 149 Harley Street at the north east corner of the block.

By 31 May, all seven clinical floors were occupied; the youngest patient to undergo elective surgery was aged three months and needed surgical repair of a hare lip. The seventh floor was the maternity ward, where the first baby, a boy, was born on 30 April to Mr and Mrs Cyril Drummond of 33 Eccleston

Beginnings **15**

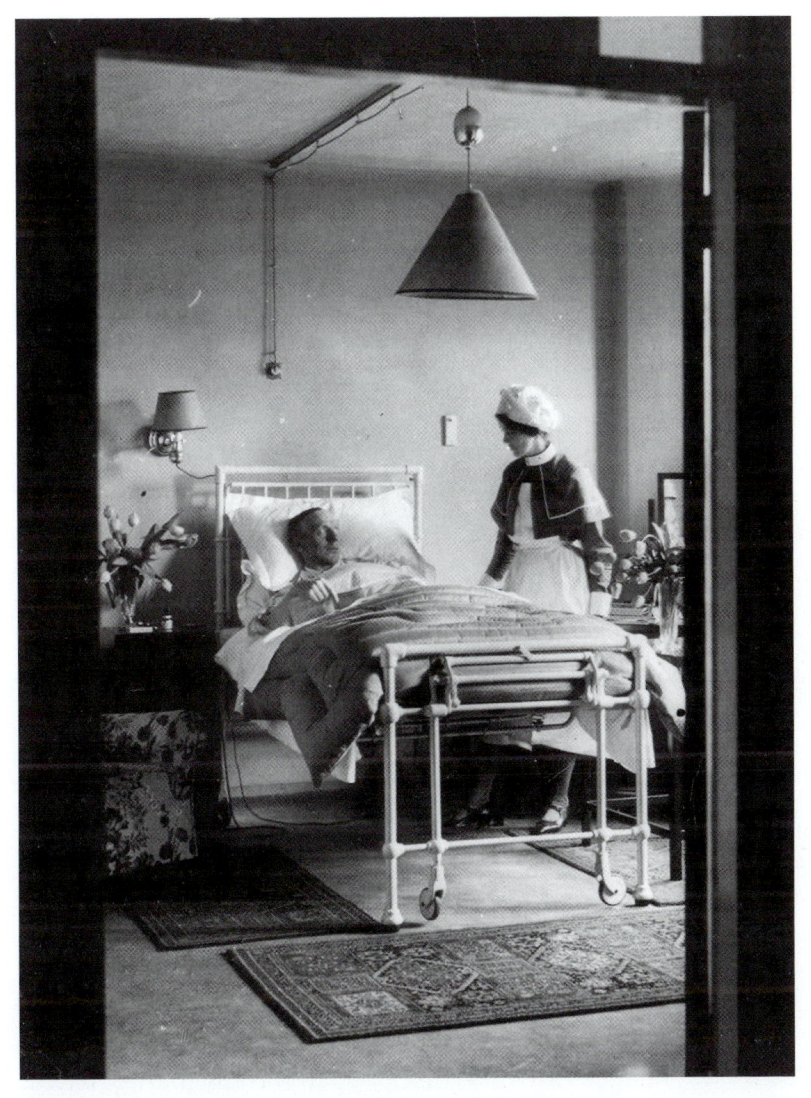

Figure 2.5 *Patient and original bedroom. Note sisters uniform with cape, long sleeves and cuffs (compare with nurses uniform in Figures 9.3 and 9.4).*

Square, SW1. The first patient to die did so, after a colectomy, on 23 February 1932 – just five days after the official opening. This confirms that, from the start, the Clinic was regarded as a hospital for major cases rather than merely a nursing home. A happier event took place in 1935 – the first set of twins, daughters for Alice and Roger Makins (subsequently our Ambassador in Washington).

3
Buildings

The site to be developed was irregular, with a frontage to the north on Marylebone Road that had angles oblique with Devonshire Place and Harley Street. The problem of this oblique frontage was solved by having four steps in the façade that faced Marylebone Road (Figures 3.1 and 3.12). This is much like Grosvenor House in Park Lane, and I believe that this prestigious building, which was completed in 1928, may well have

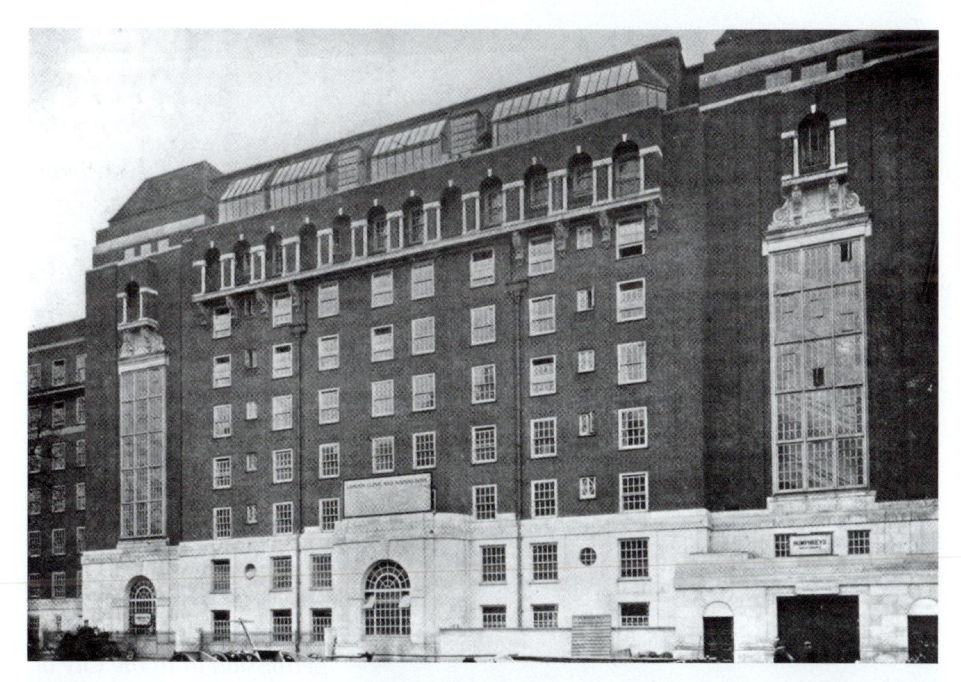

Figure 3.1 *The Marylebone Road frontage. Note operating theatre windows on top floor.*

been the inspiration for the Clinic's architect. Squat towers at either end of the main block enabled the façades on Harley Street and Devonshire Place to be lower, in order to meet planning constraints. The other buildings in the streets were therefore not dwarfed by the new development.

Figure 3.2 shows the buildings at the top of Devonshire Place before the Clinic was built, and Figure 3.3 shows the top of Harley Street and the entrance to the garden that occupied the site before 149 Harley Street was developed. The lower buildings to the north of 145 ultimately became 147 and 149 and were incorporated into the eastern façade of the development. The grand and impressive entrance through a forecourt to 149 itself is shown in Figure 3.4.

This clever design was the work of the architect CH Biddulph Pinchard, Fellow of the Royal Institute of British Architects (FRIBA). He was in his early fifties when he was commissioned to design the Clinic. He had previously been the principal architect of the Northwood Consumption Hospital and the Doctors' Clinic in Brook Street. Ten years before, he had designed the chapel and assembly room at Wellington School in Somerset. The

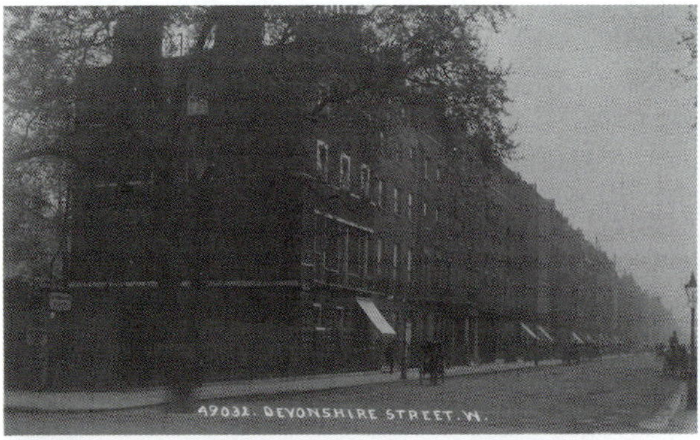

Figure 3.2 Devonshire Street, West frontage. Reproduced with kind permission from the City of Westminster Archives Centre.

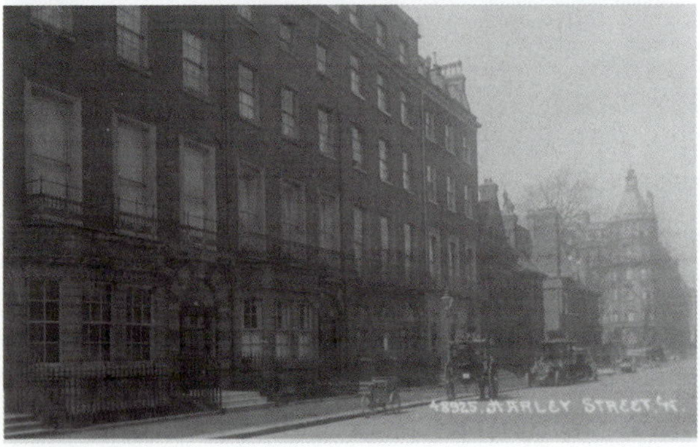

Figure 3.3 Harley Street, Northern end. Reproduced with kind permission from the City of Westminster Archives Centre.

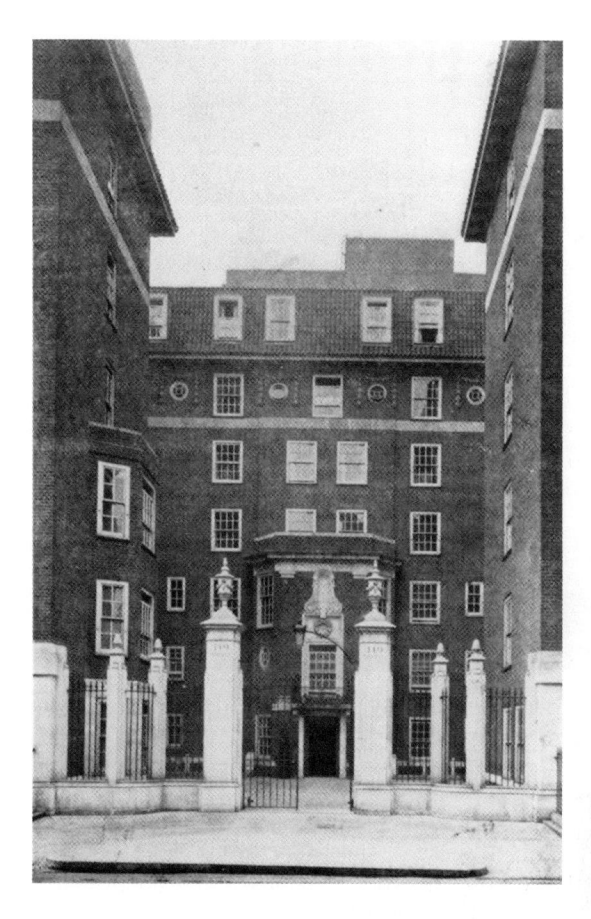

Figure 3.4 *Entrance, 149 Harley Street – unchanged to this day.*

design of the Clinic was applauded by his colleagues and praised in the architectural journal *Building Design* for having 'an air of comfort and beauty without the appearance or atmosphere of a hospital'.

The decorative architectural features outside the Clinic were made suitably opulent without being vulgar or too lavish (Figures 3.5–3.7). These were largely obscured by the London grime of peace time and the war years. They became visible again when the building was cleaned in 2001. The inside was well appointed, with pilasters and Ionic columns in the vestibule (Figure 3.8).

The specially designed furniture was of walnut and African mahogany, which was covered with cellulose for easy cleaning. Most of the rooms faced south both to capture the sun and to achieve quietness. Even in those days Marylebone Road was becoming crowded and noisy. In addition to the 214 patient rooms (Figure 3.9), which mostly had bathrooms, there were a number of suites with bedroom, sitting room and bathroom.

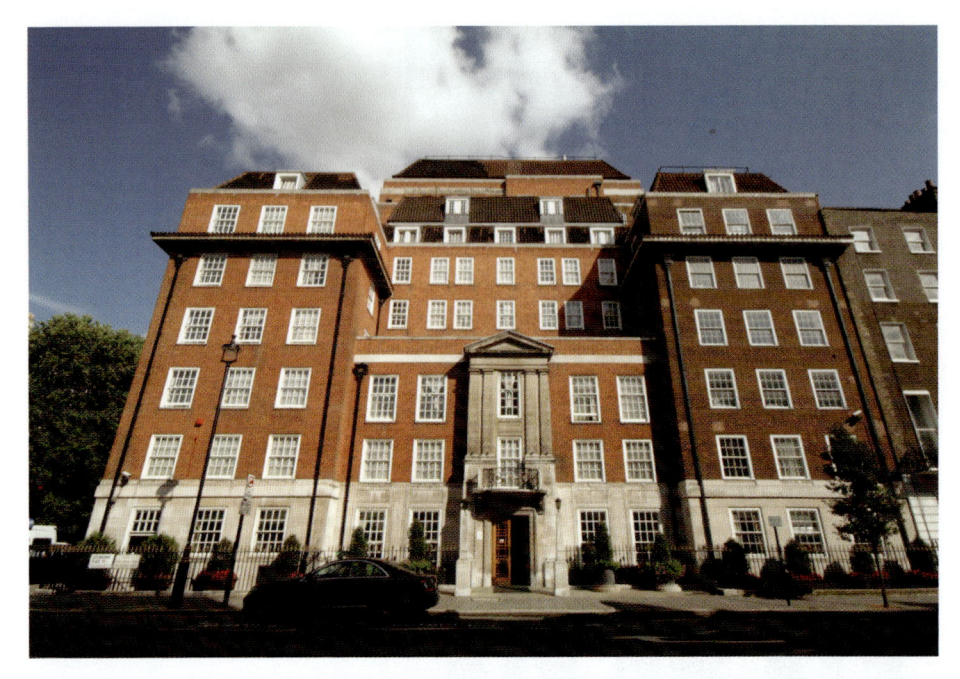

Figure 3.5 *The Devonshire Place façade can now be seen during the redevelopment of the Cancer Centre.*

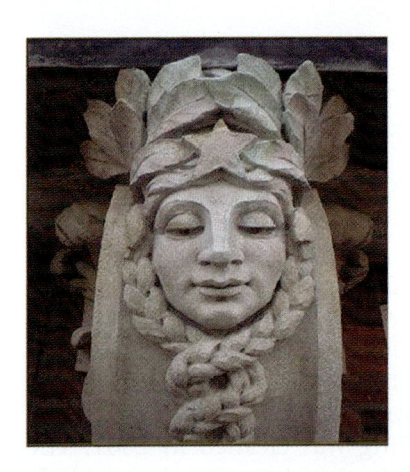

Figure 3.6 *Stone carving on north façade.*

Four floors served the needs of general cases – both surgical and medical. Other floors were allotted to specialist activities – maternity (with a terrace on the fifth floor for mothers to step out with their prams) and patients with special and dietetic needs. In addition to the main kitchen, which had electric roasting, grilling and fish-frying apparatus, were steam heaters and two gas boiling tables. The main kitchen was supplemented by a special kitchen that served those with dietetic needs.

Buildings 21

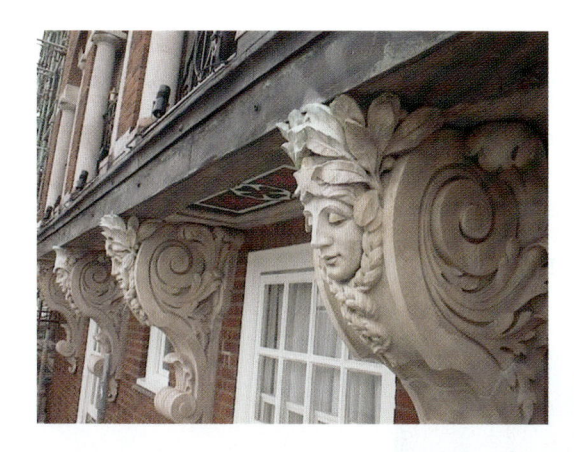

Figure 3.7 Carved stone supports on north façade.

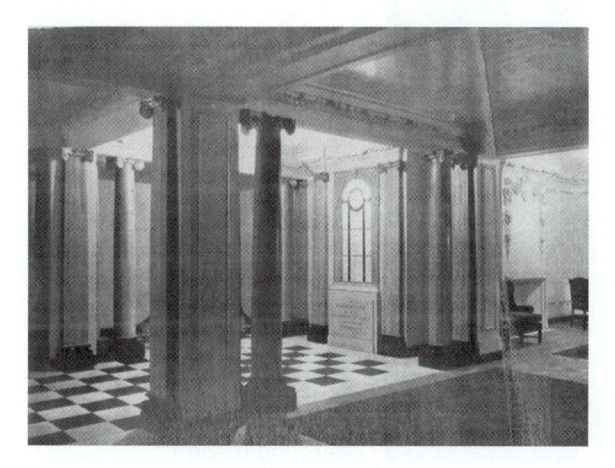

Figure 3.8 Entrance hall 20 Devonshire Place.

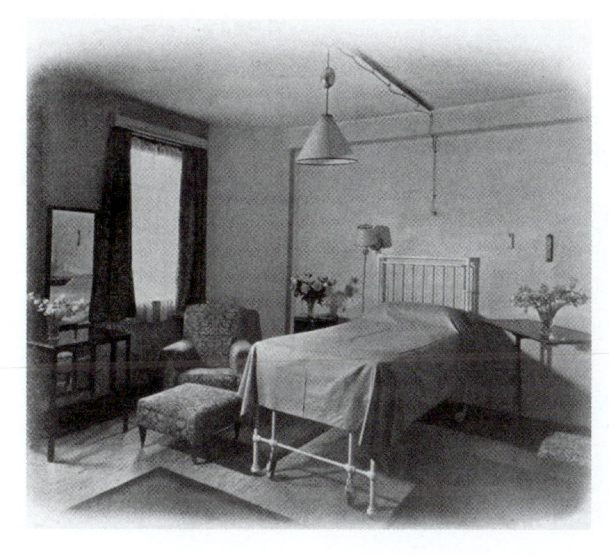

Figure 3.9 One of the original rooms.

The operating theatres were on the eighth floor. They had a north-facing light with electrically controlled blinds that could be operated by buttons within the theatre (Figure 3.10). Eight theatres in tandem were interrupted in the middle by two anaesthetic rooms. The theatre complex had sterilizing rooms on the same floor and an x-ray room and laboratory.

Throughout the hospital, a signalling system of illuminated names and lights triggered from the panel in the entrance hall was linked through the telephone exchange (Figure 3.11). This was regarded as a particularly important and novel feature.

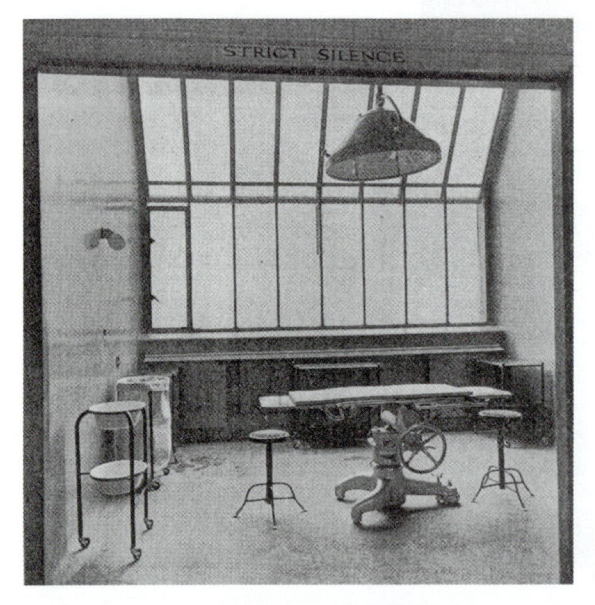

Figure 3.10 *An original operating theatre.*

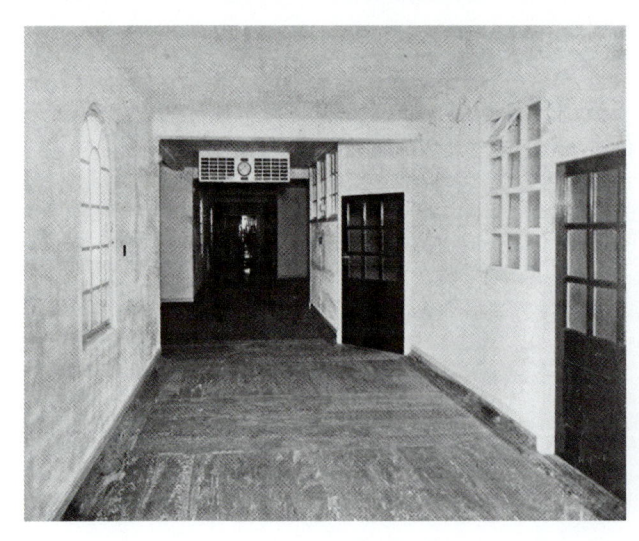

Figure 3.11 *A corridor showing the signalling system of illuminated names and lights either side of the clock.*

Buildings

Much was made of the new technology included in the building. The steel framework rested on concrete foundations that were padded with heavy felt intended to reduce both vibration and noise. In earlier days, anxiety about vibration and noise had caused much concern at University College Hospital in Gower Street and also in the consulting rooms in Harley Street. It was argued that the vibrations would interfere with the sensitive electrocardiograms and encephalograms. I think these arguments were, in fact, rather contrived in disputes about town planning proposals. These previous anxieties clearly influenced the design of the Clinic's foundations. However, I know of no evidence to suggest that the felt was or is of any practical use. An unwanted legacy of the building methods of the Clinic is the problem with any internal redevelopment. Water pipes are buried in concrete, and any noise from drilling is transmitted in every direction; up, down and horizontally. This has made the task of altering the configuration of rooms in the Clinic – essential with the changing face of medicine – expensive, noisy and difficult.

The buildings and satellites of the Clinic that our generation has inherited may well have been very different had the grandiose plans to double

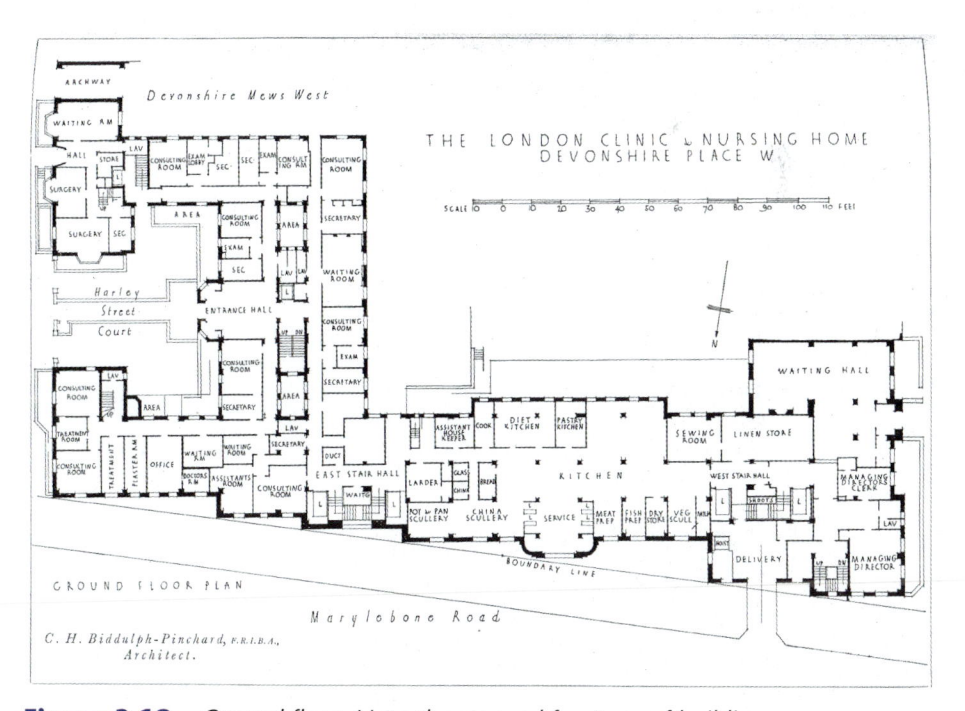

Figure 3.12 *Ground floor. Note the stepped frontage of building on Marylebone Road.*

the size of the Clinic in the 1960s (Figure 3.13) not been blocked by the preservation listing of some adjacent properties in Harley Street and Devonshire Place – as well as lack of finance.

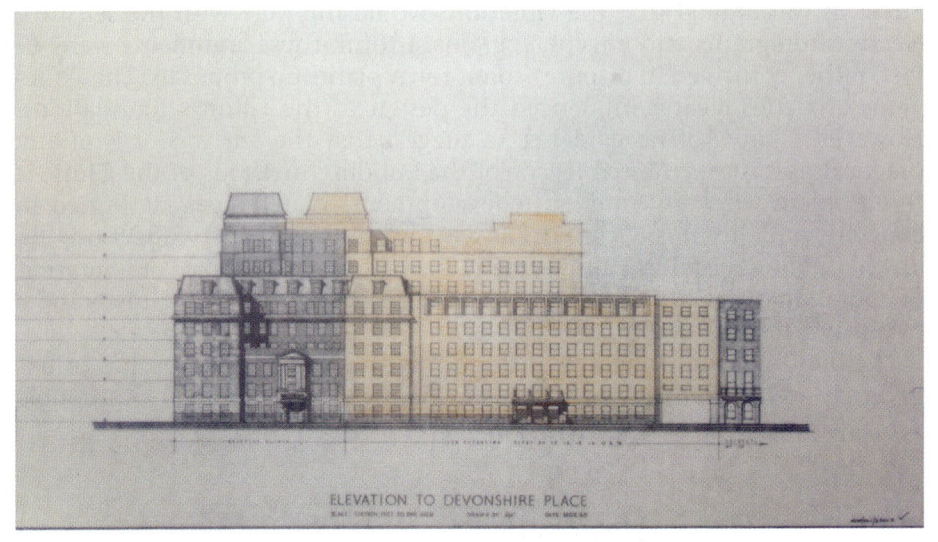

Figure 3.13 *Design for proposed 1963 development (west frontage).*

4

Top brass and general headquarters – the godlike kings of old

Those who led the board of the Clinic in the early days did so in a style characteristic of their generation. They were leaders who commanded with self-confidence and conviction; they expected to be obeyed. Inevitably, the details are somewhat clouded by time, but the members of the board seem in the words of Thomas Macauley (1800–59) to have been 'godlike kings of old'.

The Eighth Duke of Atholl was chairman of the ill-fated consortium of doctors that leased the ground from the Howard de Walden Estates in 1929 (Figure 4.1). Every inch an aristocrat, he presided over the board during the development of the site and the large overspend. He accompanied the Duke and Duchess of York at the opening ceremony in 1932. Only six months later, the receivers were called in.

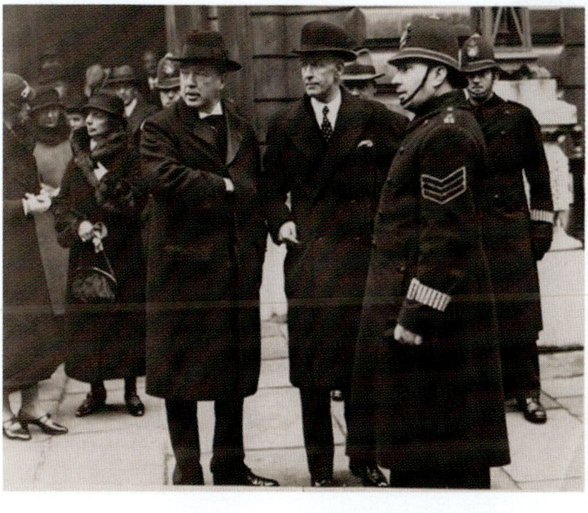

Figure 4.1 *Eighth Duke of Atholl. Seen here (on left) outside a magistrates' court when seeking permission for a sweep stake for the Derby to raise money for the Clinic before going into receivership. Reproduced with kind permission from the collection at Blair Castle, Perthshire.*

The Duke of Atholl was born in 1871. As the older son, he had the courtesy title of Lord Tullibardine and succeeded his father to the dukedom in 1917. He fought in the Royal Horse Guards at Khartoum and Atbara, winning the Distinguished Service Order (DSO), and he later saw active service in the second Boer war. He was a Conservative Member of Parliament for Perthshire and Grand Master of the Scottish Freemasons before becoming aide-de-camp to George V, a privy counsellor and Lord Chamberlain. The credentials of the first chairman seemed both impeccable and fitting for the bold venture of the Clinic. Understandably, there was dismay that it did not flourish financially at first but, fortunately, Aynsley Bridgland (later Sir Aynsley) – already associated with the project – was at hand when the receivers were called in.

Aynsley Bridgland (Figure 4.2), an Australian shipping magnate who had extensive business and real estate interests in London, was associated with the Clinic from the beginning. The receivers were called in on 24 August 1932 and Mr E Furnival Jones was appointed receiver and manager of the company's business. The winding-up order had been made on 22 June after a petition by Harrods Limited, creditors for £3,496. The Duke of Atholl, chairman, was unable to present at this meeting by reason of indisposition. It was agreed that there was no possibility of creditors receiving any dividends. Aynsley Bridgland ultimately was responsible for the formation of a company limited by guarantee and without share capital. It was called The London Clinic Limited, and it had the charitable objective of ensuring that any profit was applied to promote the clinical activities of the Clinic. The

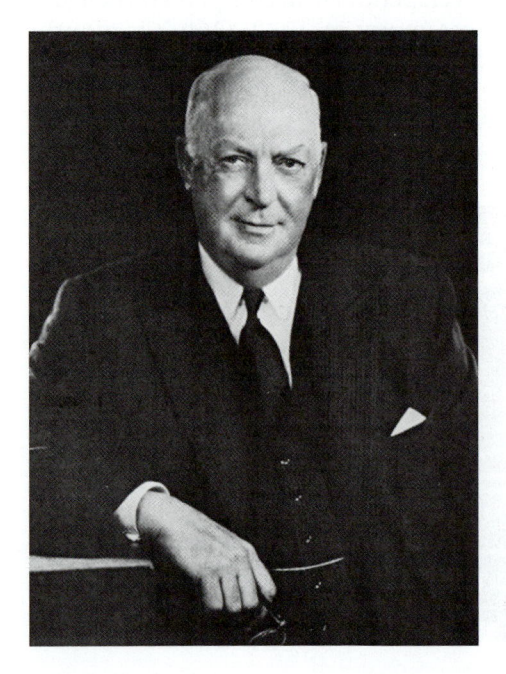

Figure 4.2 *Sir Aynsley Bridgland. Reproduced with kind permission from* The London Clinic Medical Journal 1966; **7**: 15–18.

memorandum and articles of association of this new company were incorporated on 28 November 1935 by Linklaters and Paines with seven trustees.

The letter of 24 August 1932 to the original board, which informed them that a receiver had been appointed, must have been a bitter blow. A letter to the shareholders followed, as well as a letter dispensing with the matron's services. Exchanges then followed about releasing her without greatly damaging her future career. A compromise was agreed: if she wrote a letter to say that she did not wish to continue under the receivership, she would receive one month's salary.

Initially, 175,000 shares worth £1 were issued and £180,000 mortgage money was obtained from the Equity and Law Life Assurance Society, with the builders Messrs Humphreys Ltd providing temporary finance pending completion of this mortgage. The Clinic continued to function until the receivership was terminated and the Clinic was acquired by a new company on 28 November 1935. This followed a hearing before Mr Justice Maugham in the Chancery Division on 21 February 1933, in which it was decided that the business should be sold as a going concern. This new venture was financed by the National Provincial Bank (£260,000) and Messrs Humphreys Ltd (£75,000) by Mortgage Debenture. It was agreed that the interest on this money would be paid out of any profits and that, after this charge had been met, the whole of the profits would then be applied to a reduction in the capital. This scheme was to allow Sir Aynsley Bridgland the opportunity, over time, of retrieving the personal funds that he had invested in Humphreys Ltd (building contractors of the Clinic). This obviously carried a risk to those who had invested in the project, but it was the only way forward if the Clinic was going to continue. The new company 'Trustees of The London Clinic Ltd', which had no shareholders, became a charity – and has continued as such ever since (Appendix 6).

Aynsley Bridgland had three declared ambitions when he came to England. He achieved all three. The first was to become a millionaire – which he did as a property developer. He was a member of the board of Humphreys for some years and became chairman. When he stood down from Humphreys in 1965, his place was taken by Sir Tom Hickinbotham. His second ambition was to play golf to 'scratch,' which he somehow managed by buying Prince's Golf Club, Sandwich. The final ambition was to be knighted, which he achieved by rescuing the Clinic financially and forming it into the charity of which he became chairman.

Thirty-one years later, Aynsley Bridgland, while still Chairman of the trustees, entered the Clinic as a patient himself. He paid his bills in full – as he had done over the years for the employees of the various companies with which he was involved – as he felt that 'the nursing and treatment were so good that patients returned to fitness in half the time it might take at another hospital'. Trustees, specialists and staff are still happy to commit themselves to the care and comfort of the Clinic – a fitting testimony to the original vision and the legacy of Aynsley Bridgland.

We have, of late, grown accustomed to entrepreneurs from the Antipodes. Their success results in part from a lack of prejudice leavened with hard work and over-riding self confidence. Sometimes they excel in the world of media and information technology, sometimes in property, but always there is a focus and often a ruthless streak. This was necessary when the ambitious Aynsley Bridgland came to the rescue of the Clinic with fame and fortune in his sights.

Born in Adelaide, South Australia, in 1893, Bridgland was educated at University High School, Melbourne, and subsequently went to Adelaide University. He came to Europe to prove himself in a way that was impossible at that time in Australia, and he continued with a great diversity of interests until his death in 1966. I was able to witness a similar determination in Kerry Packer, in 1940 with whom I found myself a classmate in Australia when I arrived as an evacuee from the Far East at the start of hostilities.

The diversity of Aynsley Bridgland's success included numerous property and investment trusts, but his lasting memorial undoubtedly is The London Clinic. To achieve this, he had to be confidently in control – sometimes to the dismay of the clinicians, who felt there was not enough communication between them and the administration. Bad balance sheets, however, not only require an injection of capital but also strong and somewhat ruthless management. With his background, Bridgland was able to provide these to reverse the slide to bankruptcy that ultimately would have killed what had initially been a visionary project. Without doubt, we owe the present existence of the Clinic to Aynsley Bridgland – which would give him enormous pleasure alongside his love of the golf course.

When Sir Aynsley stood down as chairman of the board of governors in 1966, he was followed by Vincent Alpe Grantham (Figure 4.3), who held office for only two years, dying after a short illness in 1968. He had been an active board member since 1936, so he was an obvious choice for chairman – especially as he had helped Bridgland save and restructure the Clinic when the receivers had been called in.

At the age of 21, adventure had enticed Grantham to Bombay to serve with Forbes, Forbes, Campbell and Company, who had originally come to prominence financing Clive of India. He later served on the Bombay Legislative Council. When he returned to England, he was chairman of the Chartered Bank and founded the Overseas Bankers Club. In addition to the Clinic, his medical interests included serving on the boards of governors of the London Chest Hospital and Brompton Hospital.

Sir Tom Hickinbotham (Figure 4.4), having been a member of the board since 1959, succeeded Grantham as chairman in 1968 and served until 1978. He had entered the Indian army in 1923, seeing action on the northwest frontier a year later and then transferring to the Indian political service before moving to the Middle East. He was governor of the Protectorate of Aden from 1951 to 1956. In his time, upgrading of the patients' rooms started and the seeds of the plan to incorporate the somewhat dilapidated

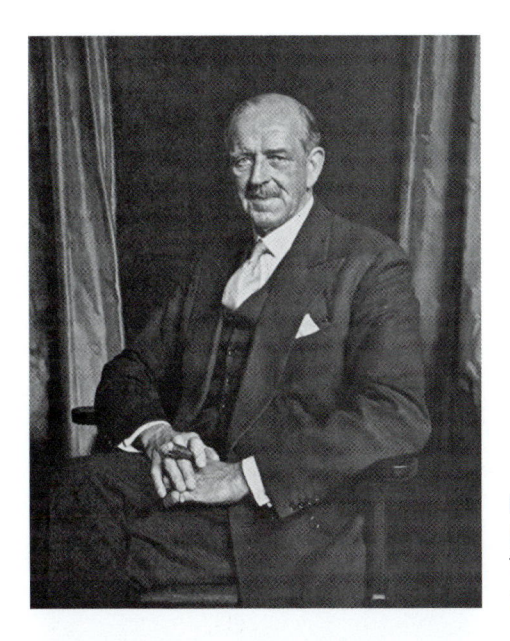

Figure 4.3 *Vincent Alpe Grantham. Reproduced with kind permission from The London Clinic Medical Journal 1969; **10**: 14–15.*

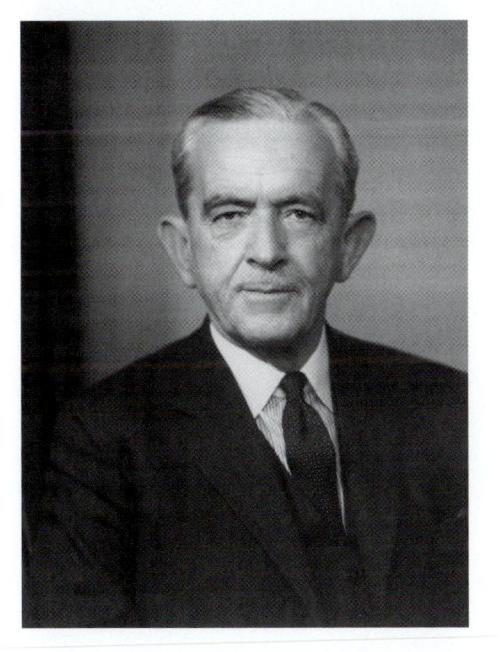

Figure 4.4 *Sir Tom Hickinbotham. Reproduced with permission from the National Portrait Gallery. NPG x82837 by Elliot and Fry, quarter plate negative, 7 December 1960.*

property at 18 Devonshire Place into the Clinic were sown. The extra space was needed to house physiotherapy, pathology and a flat for the resident medical officer.

5

Ranfurly and Ramsden years

The impeccable Sixth Earl Ranfurly (Figure 5.1) joined the board in 1969, becoming chairman from 1978 until he stepped down in 1984.

In his earlier life he was a member of Lloyds, had been chairman of Inchcape Insurance Holdings and was involved in a number of activities including the London Scout Council and Shaftesbury Homes. Most importantly, he served as governor of the Bahamas. The Clinic was nicely situated for him between Madame Tussauds and White's Club (he was chairman of both). With his wife, he started the Ranfurly Library Service, which distributed second-hand books to developing countries. When I started at the clinic in 1976, this charity was still supported by colleagues.

Lord Ranfurly visited the clinic on a Wednesday – probably between Madame Tussauds and luncheon at White's. This established a tradition that

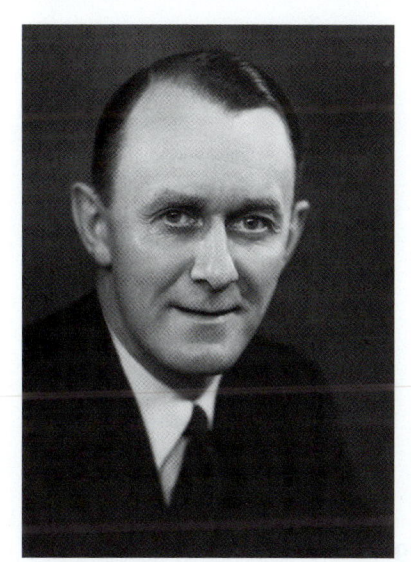

Figure 5.1 *Thomas Daniel Knox, Sixth Earl of Ranfurly. © National Portrait Gallery, London; NPG x91078 by Elliott and Fry, vintage print, 19 March 1958.*

has continued up to the present day, not only for administrative business between the chairman and the chief executive but also for board meetings.

In Lord Ranfurly's time there was a modest remuneration for members of the board, which was abolished by his successor as chairman, James Ramsden, who felt that such remuneration was inappropriate for trustees of a charity. At the time, the letter informing trustees of this change was misread by a new trustee, who immediately sent a cheque, equivalent to the previous remuneration, to the chairman. He thought it was his 'fine' for becoming a trustee of the best medical club in England (if not Europe). In earlier times, when William Hogarth became a governor of St Bartholomew's Hospital, he was so impecunious that he could not afford to pay the 'governor's fine'. He simply painted some murals (including the Pool of Bethedsa), which is now a national treasure.

Board meetings at this time had a certain informality and did not venture into such difficult topics as governance and board development. Once when a senior member of the board noticed a button missing on the waistcoat of a new board member (James Ramsden), he was able to persuade the matron to give him a needle and thread, which she carried tucked into her apron, and sewed on the button. This, of course, was in the days when matrons still wore aprons and also in the days when it was permissible to smoke a pipe at board meetings before the anti-nicotine zealots took charge of the Western world.

Michael Jenner (Figure 5.2), who was appointed deputy house governor in 1969, subsequently became house governor in 1973. At this time, he

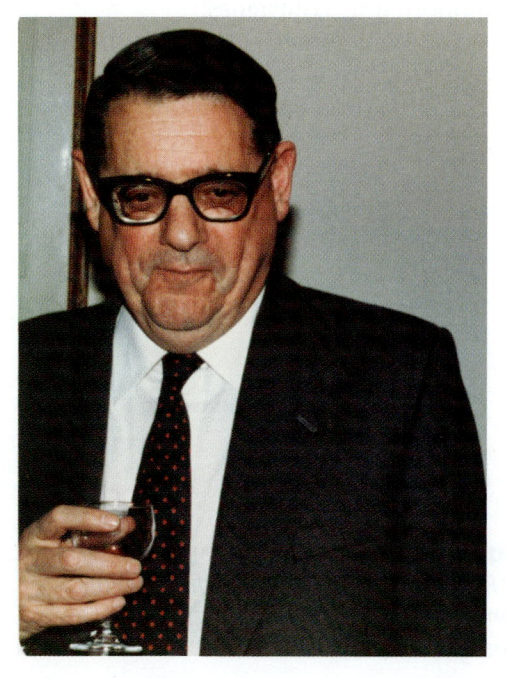

Figure 5.2 *Michael Jenner.*

found himself bridging the gap between the old guard under the leadership of Sir Tom Hickinbotham and the Ranfurly–Ramsden era. Twice a year, the governors were joined by two senior clinicians to form an executive council. This supplemented a monthly meeting of the so-called house committee, when a governor (for many years James Ramsden) met with a representative group of clinicians and the matron. Included in their number were Sir Ronald Bodley-Scott and Sir Francis Avery Jones, who had his rooms in number 149 and was the doyen of gastroenterologists until his death in 1998.

Jenner's appointment coincided not only with a long project that started upgrading patients' rooms but also the purchase of the next-door property in Devonshire Place (Number 18). For many years, this had served as a nurses' home and was in need of repair. Until now, the use of this property had been governed by terms set out in a letter of 27 August 1930 from the Howard de Walden Estate. A 'change of use' was required so that the building could become a pathology and physiotherapy department and a flat for the resident medical officers. The new lease was to run for 94 years and three months, and the development would allow the first floor of the main block to be turned into income-generating patient rooms. Relocation of the theatres from the eighth floor to the basement similarly allowed the construction of penthouse rooms for patients, further benefiting cash flow. Hand-in-hand with such changes, a new and greatly enlarged water tank was incorporated in the tower at the east of the building, which had to be raised – indeed this was achieved with great sympathy for the original design. In addition, a new lift, new boilers and much rewiring was installed, so that the Clinic was able to accommodate the predicted influx of the well-to-do of our own country and the Middle East, who by this time had discovered Harley Street. It perhaps would be true to say that Harley Street, demonstrating a new business enlightenment, had discovered the Middle East.

After the constructive dismissal, on the grounds of age, of a trustee who was giving trouble, all the governors agreed in May 1984 that they should retire at the age of 72 years. This has just been increased to 73 to allow continuity of the present chairman and board during the large ongoing developments. To meet the needs of clinical accountability, in addition to the board, a committee of senior consultants was formed. They gave advice in return for free medical treatment for themselves and their spouses. In today's terms, this was a considerable recompense for aging advisors, before youth put its hand on the tiller, with younger members on both the board and advisory committees! The practice no longer continues.

The main dialogue between the board and those engaged in clinical work – principally those with rooms in the consulting suite block that faces Harley Street (149) – was the house committee, with the chairman of the Clinic taking charge. In time, this responsibility was shared with a senior consultant. In addition to routine business and information about bed occupancy, the 'waiting list' of consultants deemed worthy of joining the select band in 149 Harley Street was considered. Due regard was paid to keeping a balance of specialities so that internal referrals could be made and the Clinic could be seen to provide a complete service. Just like the Garrick, the waiting time was some 12 or more years for popular specialities. The number of licence holders was strictly controlled by the Howard de Walden Trustees, so that the exclusive caché attached to a Harley Street practice was not debased.

Lord Ranfurly was replaced as chairman by the Right Honourable James Ramsden (Figure 5.3) in 1984. During the war, he had served with the Rifle Brigade in North-West Europe. From 1954 until 1974, he was the Conservative Member of Parliament for Harrogate and during this time was Secretary of State for War and Minister of Defence for the Army. After his parliamentary career, he became deputy chairman of the Prudential Corporation.

The house committee provided a conduit for change in clinical services. The need for an intensive therapy unit to provide suitable support for the increasingly complex clinical procedures that were being introduced was recognized. Later on, the need for a day surgery unit was considered, and this was achieved when Malcolm Miller arrived. He had already had experience setting one up with British United Provident Association (BUPA). Both projects were on the wish list inherited by the new chairman.

Not long after taking the reins as chairman, James Ramsden became a patient himself on the newly refurbished eighth floor. I well recall seeing

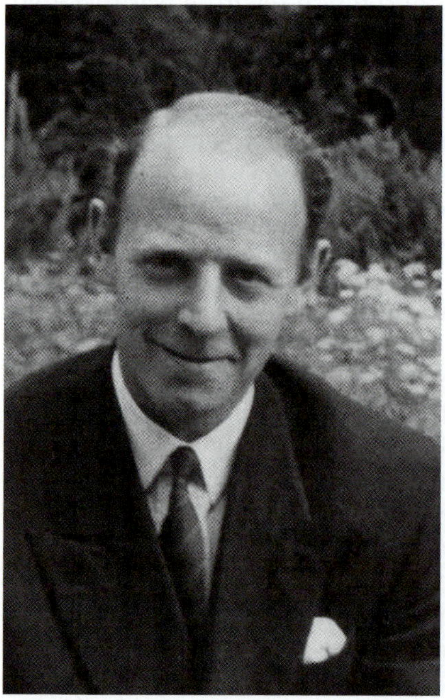

Figure 5.3 *James Ramsden.*

him (after a comparatively minor operation) perambulating around the corridors in his dressing gown. Naturally I thought he was reducing the possibility of a deep vein thrombosis. He was, however, networking between patients – among their number was John Paul Getty II (Figure 5.4), who was a long-stay patient who had become somewhat reclusive after a series of misfortunes. He shared a love of Sherlock Holmes with James Ramsden, and he was himself rather like Holmes' character 'the persistent patient'. Getty's special relationship with the Clinic during his prolonged sojourn cannot be better expressed than by the fact that his dog, together with that of the house governor, was allowed up the back stairs to visit him.

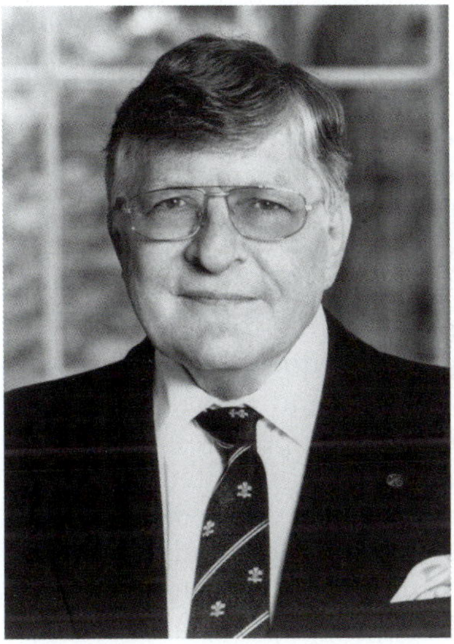

Figure 5.4 *Sir Paul Getty.*

As the friendship between the convalescent chairman, James Ramsden, and John Paul Getty II blossomed, there was an exchange of gifts. Getty's presentation to the new chairman was a bottle from the vineyard of CM Rothschild (notable vintage and numbered bottle). The chairman's gift was a book by Lord Nutsford, which gave an account of raising money for a London Hospital – not a particularly subtle form of subliminal programming – but it worked. Getty's reawakening interest in life proved to be the spring of a summer of charitable bequests from which the Clinic was destined to benefit. Husbanding this benefaction was a letter written by Lord Lloyd (Geoffrey Lloyd, MP) who was a patient in the room next to Getty's. This letter detailed a tax-efficient method of charitable giving – even for an American citizen, as Getty then was.

In the meantime, Christopher Gibbs – brother of a board member, Roger (later Sir Roger) Gibbs, who was chairman of the Howard de Walden Estates, and a friend of Getty – did some figures. To put the Clinic on its feet and buy the freehold from the Howard de Walden Trustees (which they were unlikely ever to have agreed to sell) was estimated to cost £40m. In the end, a generous donation of £2m was received from Getty to fund the intensive therapy unit and hydrotherapy unit. This deal was, in many ways, the result of the devoted attention Getty had received from all the Clinic's staff. Among them can be identified Ros Yearly, the physiotherapist, Paul Christoforou, the ubiquitous messenger and humorist, Andrew Holmes, who was skilful in fixing Getty's gadgets and finally the Scottish sister who gave direct orders, "Turn over Mr Getty, I want to rub your bum." Such a down-to-earth relationship leavened by the care and devotion of the Clinic had yielded rewards. Although not exactly bailing the Clinic out of its financial problems, the gift was able to pump-prime recovery by giving facilities that would enable the provision of up-to-date services that themselves fed happily into the improving income stream.

The debt owed to Paul Getty is recognized and commemorated in a way that is both subtle and enduring. A sculpture by Lady Bacon in a niche over the door of number 149 (which is destined to become the main entrance of the Clinic) gives a benediction to all who enter (Figure 5.5). The snake – a symbol of medicine and regeneration – had symbolically come out of a fire and 'bitten the hand' of Paul Getty.[1] This persuaded him to concentrate his mind on the Clinic and resulted in the generous bequest. The hand with three fingers extended represents the Holy Trinity, and it makes a strong statement, in bronze, of the ethos of the Clinic and hopefully a message of salvation to all those who enter. Alas the spikes that represented the flames of the bonfire were lost recently when the building was cleaned.

In absolute terms, the injection of capital that enabled the development of two of the requirements for up-to-date clinical care (an intensive treatment unit and a hydrotherapy unit), while being a start, is small in today's terms. The timing was important, however, and it acted as a catalyst to raise morale and make the Clinic believe in its potential. Endoscopy and day sur-

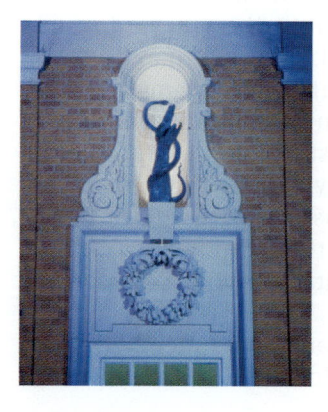

Figure 5.5 *Sculpture in niche, 149 Courtyard, by Lady Bacon (see Figure A9.4).*

gery units were to follow in due course. The contemplative, pipe-smoking chairman James Ramsden was laying the foundations for the future. Little could he have realized that the efficient financial control that was to be introduced by his successor would rapidly increase this figure over a year or two by a factor of three. Profits generated by the Clinic would, in the future, fund developments.

Although bed occupancy was improving, this was not yet backed up by sufficiently strict credit control, adequate pricing and accurate billing. This was merely good business practice, which had, over the years, not really been thought to go hand-in-hand with a caring profession. The world was changing, however, while the overdraft was growing. The need for the Clinic to be run on a strictly economic basis actually had been identified by Peat-Marwick-Mitchell in a memorandum to the governors in 1939. This lesson had to be relearned to allow survival and meet increasing competition from other institutions, including private wings of NHS hospitals. Private hospitals had to sing from the same hymn sheet as the public sector. The providers of private medical insurance were also experiencing their own financial problems.

In 1981, Richard (Dick) J Kent (Figure 5.6) followed Mr Michael Jenner as house governor. He brought with him years of experience from a similar position at the Royal Marsden Hospital. He was a patient, kind and conscientious team player, as one would expect from his days in the army, merchant navy and on the rugby field. His understanding of human nature enabled him to communicate, motivate and engender loyalty. The increasing formality of committees and lines of reporting, however, was appearing on the horizon. Before it finally overtook us, his succinct minutes drafted in bold long-hand sufficed. I hope some are preserved to show how things were done at that time!

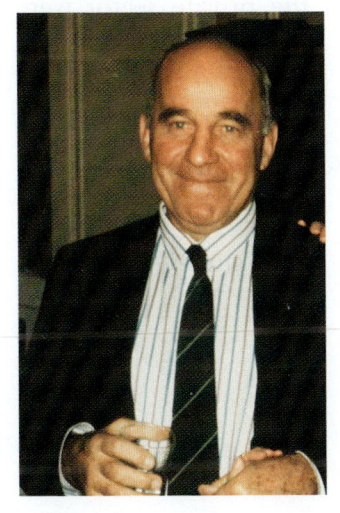

Figure 5.6   *Richard (Dick) J Kent*

Since the upgrading of the rooms when Mr Jenner had been appointed house governor in 1973, little had been done to the fabric of the building. The requirements and expectations of patients for en-suite bathrooms and other luxuries had increased. Very little money had been put aside for further refurbishment, partly because the Clinic was the victim of its own success and there was reluctance to take rooms out of service for upgrading. In addition, putting money aside for the upgrading of rooms was thought, to some extent, to be a conflict between creature comforts and the Clinic's charitable status.

James Ramsden felt that he had a very good in-house team in the estates department which was involved in the refurbishment work. This certainly was the case and they were well led and directed by Tony Beecroft and Kevin Goodbun. The opportunities for refurbishment and the development of the buildings were a challenge that has allowed this powerful duo to find their full potential. The Clinic has benefited by having such a strong team. The space they have developed throughout the Clinic is elegant, welcoming and fits the clinical needs well. Their legacy will remain and be a happy working environment for many years. The pathology outpatients department was awarded the International Design Effectiveness Award 2001–02 in the category of 'Interiors – office and commercial'. Overseeing the present expansion of the Clinic's quantum leap and coordinating the project is Paul Wood, Strategy Director.

A lot was achieved at this time – a difficult period – which was heavily dependent on the loyalty, contribution and sense of community spirit that pervaded throughout the staff. Clinical, nursing, administrative staff and the whole backbone of the establishment – from the head porter and the theatre technicians to the estates department – were involved.

The projects addressed at this time are worth listing, because they underpinned the successful first inspection and certification of a private hospital by the Kings Fund when the highest marks in the private sector were achieved in 1999:

- refashioned front hall
- education department
- endoscopy unit, with equipment by KeyMed (Medical & Industrial Equipment) Ltd
- minimally invasive treatment unit (MITU)
- installation of magnetic resonance imaging (MRI) (initially franchised out to a consortium)
- new pharmacy
- oncology unit
- physiotherapy and hydrotherapy pool
- refurbishment of patients' rooms
- staff dining room
- terrace restaurant for patients.

No wonder BUPA expressed an interest in buying the Clinic.

My generation of consultants was perhaps somewhat dismissive about institutions such as business schools and the ideas that they disseminated, including cash flow, human resources and personnel management. To be able to think objectively and rationally about the delivery of healthcare, is essential in both the public and private sectors. Such ideas could not be put in place immediately, and the new chairman, James Ramsden, clearly believed that time spent in reconnaissance was never wasted. For him this started when he was a patient, and it continued after his recovery, with his sleeping three nights a week on a temporary bed in the board room – rather like Winston Churchill in the cabinet's war rooms. He was not elephantine in his appearance, but he was a good listener, he never forgot and the gestation period before he was able to set the scene for the future was, like the elephant's, about four years. In order to help him in his endeavours, he brought Michael Abrahams, a shrewd and persuasive businessman, onto the board. He was instrumental in finding a deputy for Dick Kent in the form of Malcolm Miller, an accountant from BUPA.

The committee's structure was changed when the new chairman formed the medical advisory committee (MAC), which had greater consultant representation (see Appendix 5). I well remember going through the bed occupancy and cash flow at our meetings each month. One or occasionally two board members were present. All could come but they had many outside commitments, which made regular attendance impossible. What concerned me with this committee, and indeed the committees that succeeded it, was that the Chairman reported to himself and the board, as he chaired both. No clinical representative was on the board (even in attendance), and there was no doctor on the board for many years. A curious way to run a hospital, I thought but it seemed to work and things should not change quickly but should simply evolve. After some years of pressure, this eventually was rectified, when a retired radiotherapist, Sir Christopher Paine, was recruited. He had practised out of London and was therefore thought not to have a conflict of interest. Unlike NHS hospitals, no active clinician is ever in attendance at the Clinic's board meeting, even today.

The committee, however, did establish a far closer relationship between the Board, the administrators and the powerhouse of consultants in number 149. It served – even if temporarily – to stave off the error of excluding clinical consultants from administration that at one time crept into the NHS. Previously there had been what a disgruntled consultant in number 149 some years ago described as 'creeping fossilization...with little cross-linkage between the medical members and the administration'. The new wind-of-change was therefore welcome to dispel the apartheid that some felt had developed. It is right now for professional administrators to grapple with risk management, targets and budgets and not leave this in the hands of clinicians. There is, however, the danger that in doing so, medicine could be somewhat degraded to a service industry rather than a self-regulating profession.

Brand loyalty is a concept of modern marketing. This was rightly demanded, where practicable, from consultants who were in the favoured position of being able to have consulting rooms in 149 which had many advantages – including a very reasonable rent, or rather 'service charge'. From 1962 onwards, the minutes of the Board meetings note that consultants in 149 should be encouraged to make greater use of the facilities. Bed occupancy was fed not only by those in 149 but by others on the books of the Clinic. If they played their part in this respect, they knew that the executive could be relied on to look after the cost control and budget. This included disciplining the medical attachés and foreign embassies who were slow to settle their bills. Those who were guilty were brought into line at this time by Ian Gilmour, a friend of the Chairman, who had been a politician with a deep experience of the Middle East. He helped recover £500,000 of outstanding debts.

Reference
1. *Holy Bible*. Acts 28, verses 2–6.

6
The third way

The appointment of Michael Abrahams to the board by James Ramsden was the Clinic's 'wind of change'. From Yorkshire, Abrahams (Figure 6.1) was a neighbour of Ramsden, and the two were not only friends on and off the hunting field but respected and admired each other. Their success and experience in life had come from very different fields – Ramsden an establishment figure in Westminster, Abrahams a shrewd and suc-

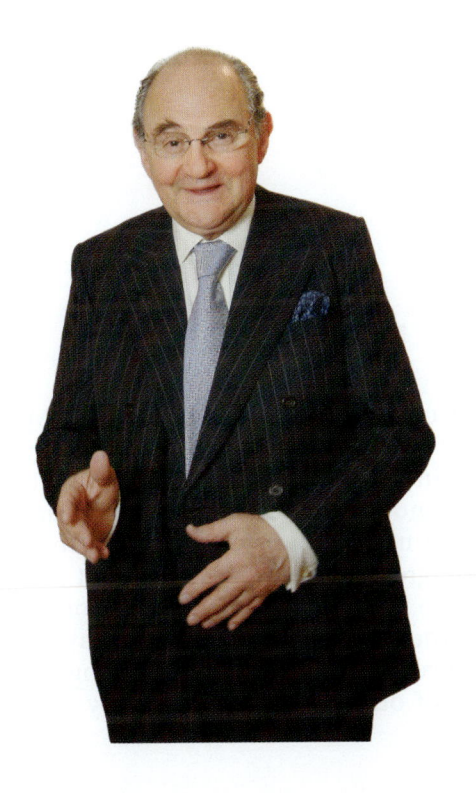

Figure 6.1   *Michael Abrahams.*

cessful figure in the City, with acknowledged business acumen. His experience ranged from textiles to insurance and from communications to national charities. He became chairman of the Clinic in April 1996. When I asked James Ramsden about the new chairman, he simply said 'Michael knows how to run things', and he has been proved right.

One of Abraham's first acts after his appointment to the Board was to recruit Malcolm Miller (Figure 6.2) from BUPA as assistant to Dick Kent. When initially interviewed for the job, Malcolm Miller was asked how soon he expected to be able to pay off the mounting overdraft. Like an experienced clinician who gets used to predicting the time-course of the cure or demise of a patient, his cautious prediction of solvency was met – even with time to spare.

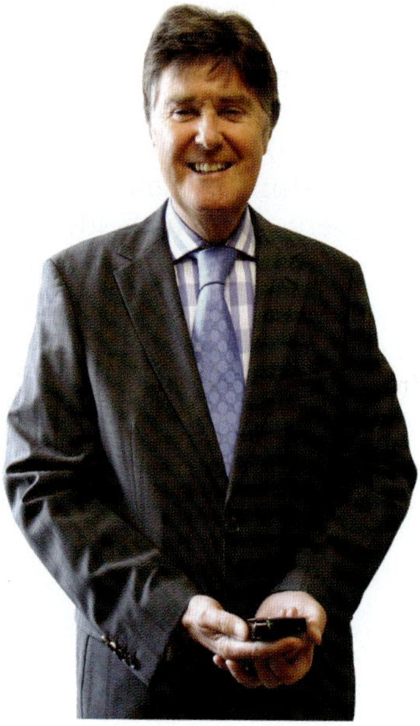

Figure 6.2 *Malcolm Miller.*

The initial period of trial by ordeal, or rather audit, placed Malcolm Miller in the happy position of having the Board's confidence to continue with the changes needed for modern business efficiency. The Clinic had been marking time financially for a while; however, modern financial management with credit control, agreed profit margins, proper budgeting and efficient billing were introduced with great effect. They were not always appreciated by the clinicians – or even the patients – who saw money-up-front as somewhat commercial. Without this, survival would have been doubtful. At the time a scarcity of private beds in London was giving way to a surplus as a result of the building of other private hospitals by UK and foreign-based insurance companies.

The international financiers and healthcare insurers were looking for other targets, and the UK was seen to provide rich pickings in a market that had rather lagged behind much of the developed world. This was undoubtedly the result of the initial excellence of the NHS, which had flourished for 25 years on the enthusiasm and goodwill of the doctors and nurses. All believed in the philosophy and social principles on which it was based. It was feeling the strain, however, and, like the railways and schools, had been starved by successive governments of cash for buildings and equipment. In addition, realistic staff development, both in numbers and financial rewards, had been neglected in a world that offered large financial rewards to many with less training.

Now, however, the need for the private sector to supplement and even work in partnership with the NHS was beginning to be accepted by the political think-tanks of both left and right. The market was there, the expertise was there and almost immediately foreign investors were there. The Clinic as the traditional English brand image had to reinvent itself in the face of competition.

When Michael Abrahams took over, the Clinic was largely run by the house governor and matron, and the committee structure was traditionally informal. The financial management and control at the best was somewhat amateur and at the worst weak. The Clinic had effectively outgrown the structure that supported it. Modern management methods had to be introduced. New wine could not be put into old bottles, and genetic modification rather than natural evolution was required. Malcolm Miller inevitably moved in the direction of an executive board. Initially, there was an executive committee with just three members – the matron, chief executive and finance director. The formation of a formal department of finance with a director led to the introduction of modern financial control, audit and strategic planning, which produced a great improvement in the financial well-being of the Clinic. The management and movement of credit days and debit and cash flow activity have enabled the Clinic to invest in leading-edge technology from revenue. When analysing patient flow, as well as cash flow, it has become evident that although the number of inpatients has fallen, those who are in the Clinic are more seriously ill. In financial jargon, this means that there is more day-patient activity and, because of a decrease in the average credit days, the revenue can be made to work more efficiently to the clinic's advantage. In summary, the Clinic's finances are more professionally and systemically regulated, enabling targets and promises to be met. The whole financial structure was more 'energized'. After a year, the executive committee metamorphosed into the executive board drawing in the new directorates that were evolving. The new departmental managers took responsibility, 'owned' their budgets and addressed management issues. Most of the loyal and dedicated old staff were able, with training, to marry their in-house experience to these new demands. A few were content to take their memories into retirement but happy to see the Clinic flourish.

Patient satisfaction became paramount, and where services were seen to be failing, remedies had to be found. In order to achieve this, the discrepancy between what was thought to be satisfactory and the reality of the situation – whether clinical or housekeeping – had to be under constant surveillance. Indeed, they were right down to the ice-making machines on the floors. These were challenging but not carefree times. Standards were raised and the need for quality recruiting addressed. National vocational qualifications (NVQs) were introduced for 'customer-facing' staff to achieve a high level of courtesy. Unlike the initial recruitment of staff, when the Clinic preferentially employed ex-servicemen, the present policy had to be to recruit the very best people who could be found for the job. In addition, it was necessary to pay the same rates that could be obtained for appointments in a more commercial field.

Supported by a competent executive board (Figure 6.3), the chairman and the chief executive, as Malcolm Miller was to be called (rather than house governor), were free to devote time to managing the strategy of change and what was to become the quest for excellence. Forming a strategy for the future – short-, medium- and long-term – was vital. This had to be addressed formally, with half of every other meeting of the executive board addressing this vital component of success.

There were clinical issues to be considered – the range of services and the numbers of specialties, the age profile of the consultants and the provision of sessional rooms. The logistical problems of the delivery of facilities with limited space and recruiting staff of all kinds were never far away. Having

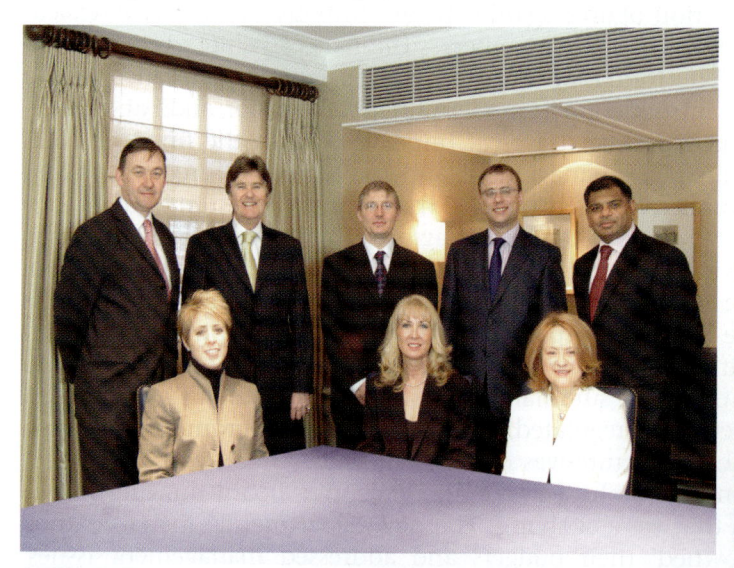

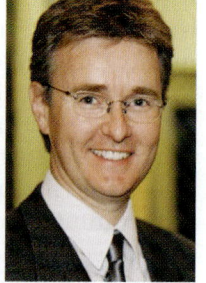

Figure 6.3 *Executive board. Back row: Mike Roberts, Malcolm Miller, Tony Beecroft, Andrew Barker, Sanjay Shah. Front row: Karen Bullivant, Amanda Hallums, Gillian Irvine. Right hand photo: Paul Wood (missing from main photograph).*

acquired staff, their training and retention required positive planning and input. There was also a need to grapple with issues such as the nationally imposed criteria of governance, which appeared from nowhere and brought with it a new concept that the chief executive was legally responsible for all clinical as well as administrative aspects. A way of going forward had to be put in place and this spawned a number of further committees, such as clinical effectiveness (which metamorphosed into governance), risk management, clinical multi-disciplinary committees, and accreditation.

Philosophical questions kept appearing on the new chairman's horizon, such as 'What is the purpose of the Clinic and to whom is the board responsible?' – certainly not to shareholders as it was a charity. He solved this conundrum to his own personal satisfaction by realizing that the members of the Board were accountable to themselves and the justification had to be to strive for excellence – that is and must ever be the accepted goal. This ethos has now been taken on by all the Clinic staff and is encapsulated in the mission statement and philosophy in Appendix 2.

The profit motive usually drives progress, even in the medical field. This is not the case as far as the Clinic is concerned, because of its charitable status. Serving the patient must be the motive. This objective – striving for the excellence of patient care – is not specific to the Clinic but fortunately has worked in a spectacular way. There are undoubtedly many factors. The whole is always greater than the sum of the parts. Somehow the parts have been conspicuously good and the sum remarkable in the short and medium term.

A series of dinner discussions with consultants were held in the Garrick (that ultimate temple of networking) to feed ideas to the chairman. These meetings were pleasurable but also important. What was less pleasurable (but necessary) for the chairman was to take on the insurance companies with whom the clinicians and hospitals (including the Clinic) were on a collision course. Undoubtedly driven by their own financial needs and the apparently bottomless pit of money required to provide effective clinical care, they had withdrawn behind defences with a confrontational and self-protective palisade. Things are different now that the insurance companies are 'customer facing' rather than confrontational. They still need to crank up and simplify their internal management and financial control and refrain from shedding some of the administrative load that they should bear themselves onto consultants' clinical secretaries.

The board of governors, in line with the charity commissioner's thinking, has become a board of trustees (Figure 6.4) with a wide mix of skills. They are able to address the need for internal financial audit, public relations and clinical issues. There is even a trustee responsible for that all important resource, nursing, which has to be husbanded carefully.

Significant developments were required, with expensive equipment such as endoscopes, monitors and scanners on the shopping list but space was at a premium. Some decisions about the long-term rationalization of services

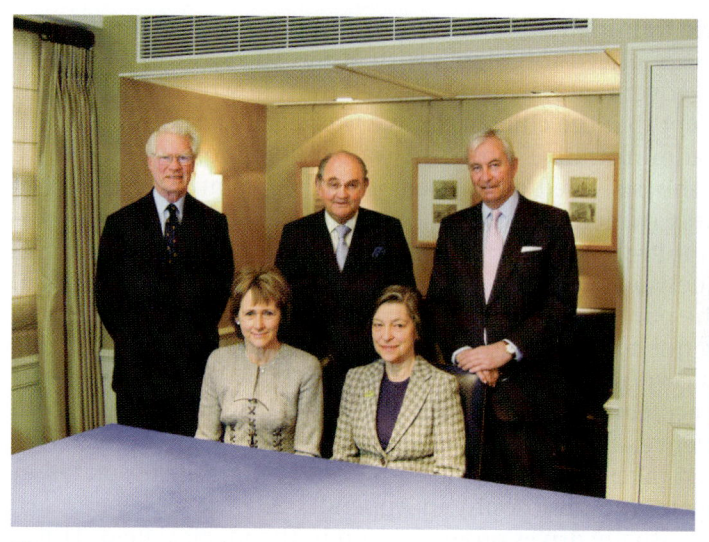

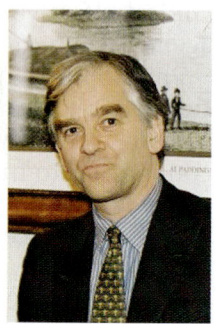

Figure 6.4 *The board of trustees. Back row: Sir Christopher Paine, Mr Michael Abrahams, Mr Richard A Hambro. Front row: Duchess of Devonshire, Lady Eccles of Moulton. Right hand photo: Rupert S Ponsonby (missing from main photograph).*

had to be undertaken – no cardiothoracic surgery, for example. Having already addressed the need for an intensive care unit, there were now other demands, which included health screening, endoscopy, scanning and pathology. All needed cash and space. Fortunately, the trend for shorter admissions and day treatment facilities – including dialysis, chemotherapy and surgery – eased some of the pressure on space. This allowed more room to be devoted to some of the newer diagnostic procedures, which were able to feed into the income stream.

Where did all of this place the Clinic? There was a feeling that we could now hold our head up high among competitors. There was understandable pride when the Clinic received the highest rating award that can be given by the King's Fund. With a successful cash-rich business, the Clinic could now develop, have the finest equipment and provide a state-of-the-art service. Those delivering healthcare have to comply with that bureaucratic dinosaur, the Department of Health in certain ways; having done that, there is no need for a deeper relationship. They are therefore free to identify and meet clinical need. The clinicians working in such a favourable environment have been able to initiate clinical advances in a way that might not have seemed possible 40 years ago when privacy and comfort were the chief aims of private nursing homes and clinics.

The nursing department has taken a notable lead in education that has helped staff motivation (Figure 6.5). This initiative has not so far been properly addressed, however, by their medical colleagues. Consultants now retire from the NHS earlier and pursue their clinical lives in comparative

The third way

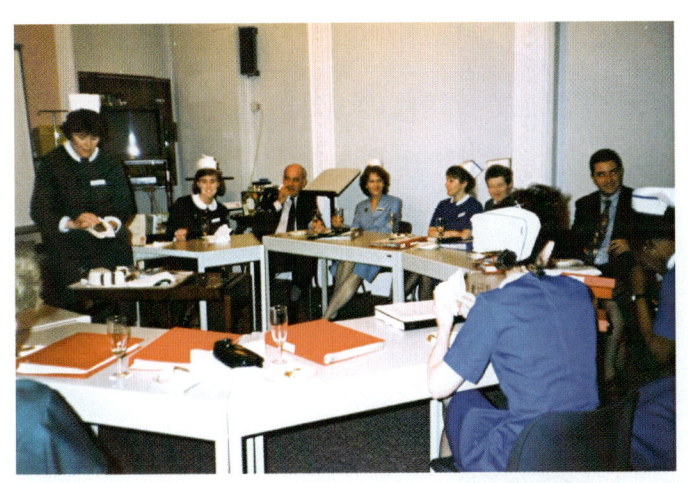

Figure 6.5 *Beginning of nurse education meetings, which coincided with the retirement of Dick Kent (third from left).*

isolation. Their continuing professional development and research will formally have to be addressed by the Clinic – perhaps linked with the multidisciplinary clinical meetings. The trend for satellite 'chambers' of specialists with similar interests is developing and these will be integrated with the Clinic. Such chambers will require a variety of services to be provided such as information technology, pathology and audit. They will carry varying obligations to use other Clinic facilities but these will not be as strong as the financially favourable 'service charge' demanded of those in 149 or the new consulting rooms in 3–5 Devonshire Place. The Clinic has to ensure, therefore, that loyalty is promoted by the excellence of the services provided.

Having put its house in order, the Clinic can now address the future and develop its services. Apart from having more clinical space with the relocation of consulting rooms to 3–5 Devonshire Place, there is the exciting prospect of having a comprehensive oncology centre across the road in Devonshire Place – embracing investigation, chemotherapy and radiotherapy. What is planned as the finest centre of its kind in the world will be linked to the main building by a tunnel under the road (Figures 6.6–6.9). This new centre, in addition to providing treatment, will always have its sights on advancing medical science and, employing the sound-bite of the day, be 'fit for purpose'.

Apart from the chairman, chief executive, his indispensable and longstanding personal assistant, Charmian Heyland, and the director of nursing and clinical services, all the directorates have moved across the Marylebone Road to Ulster Terrace. This has a fine Nash façade framed by plane trees and provides a view for those patients not favoured by having a room on

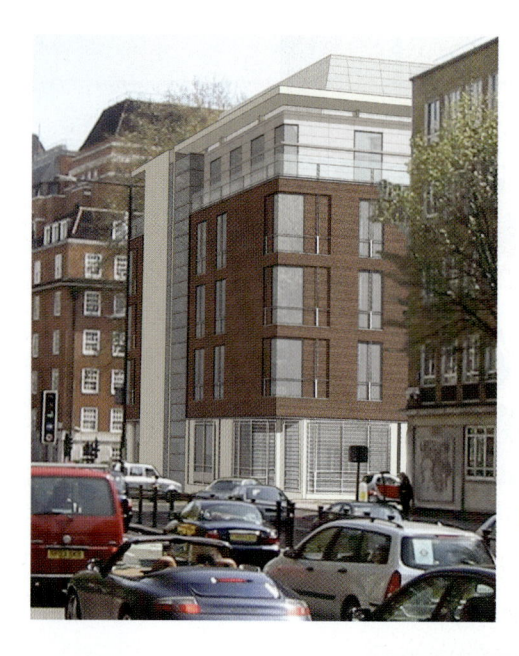

Figure 6.6 Computer-generated image of the cancer centre along the Marylebone Road adjacent to the Clinic.

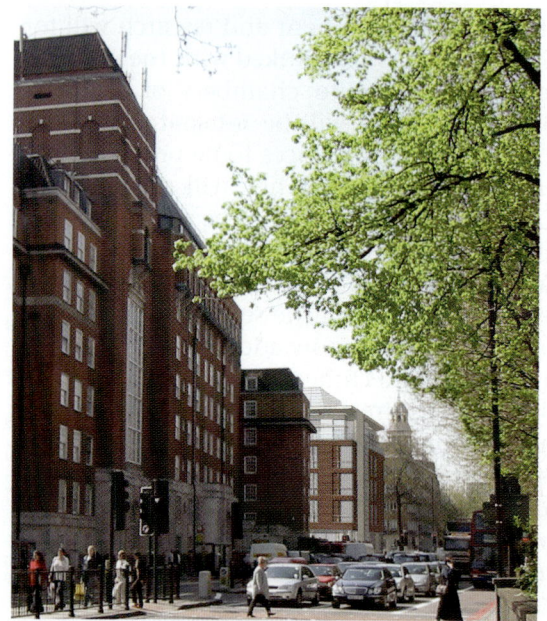

Figure 6.7 Computer-generated image of the cancer centre looking west along the Marylebone Road.

the south side of the main block. I wonder what they would think if they could actually see into the offices in Ulster Terrace, which are inhabited by staff peering at the computer screens that are required to support their admission and hopefully trouble-free progress from infirmity to health.

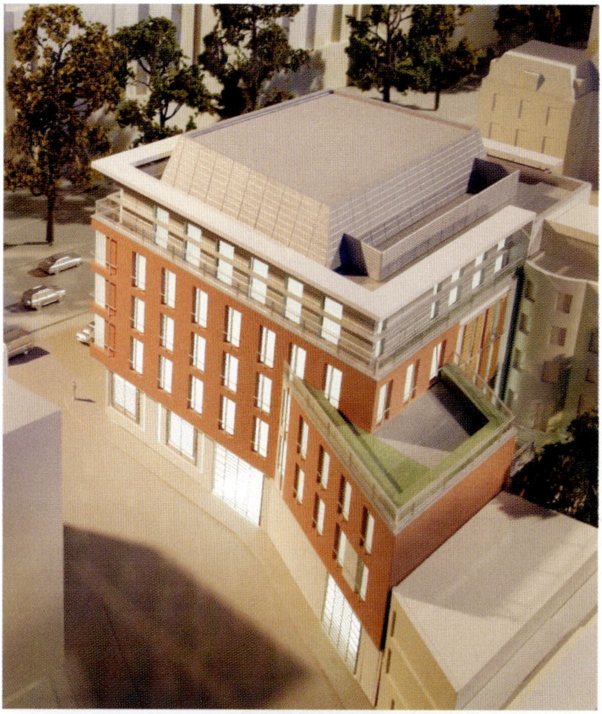

The third way 49

Figure 6.8 *Computer-generated image of the cancer centre from the south west. (See Appendix 13 for preliminary site assessment.)*

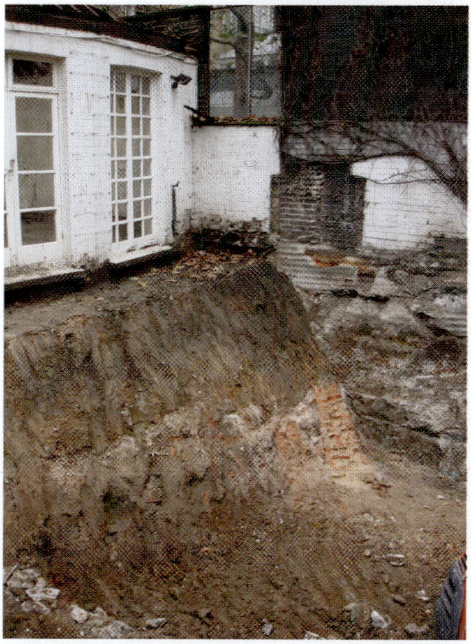

Figure 6.9 *Demolition of the site of the new development has unearthed the remains of Dove Cottage (see Appendix 14 for detail).*

The old logo that served from the foundation was replaced when Michael Abrahams became chairman. To mark the 75th anniversary, the Clinic has been rebranded with a new logo. The changes are shown below (Figure 6.10).

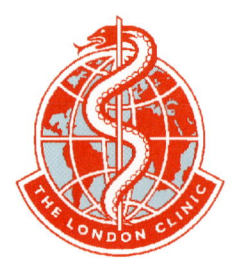

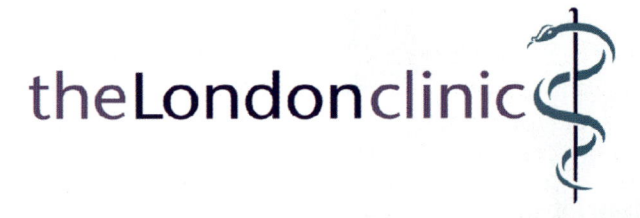

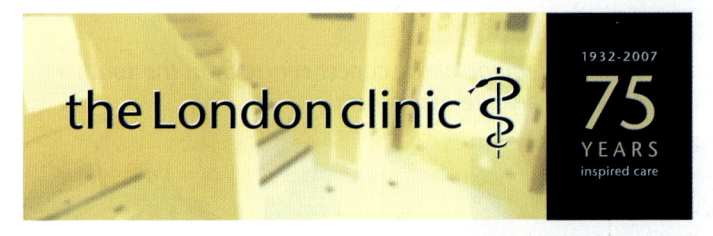

Figure 6.10   *Logos*

7
Patients

The Hippocratic Oath does not allow any distinction to be made by the physician in respect of colour, creed or social standing; so it is at the Clinic – although, of course, the ability to pay is the common denominator. The worthy middle classes with sufficient funds were from the beginning leavened by aristocrats whom the Clinic welcomed with ever-open arms. They were in turn as anxious to be seen using 'the palace of health' as they were to be seen at the opera. Inevitably, politicians from home and abroad found the quality of care and privacy appealing – and, when well enough, could order their wine from the Clinic's extensive cellar. Heads of state and royalty from home and abroad found the Clinic able to meet all their needs – including various discreet entrances distant from the prying eyes and ears of the media. A more mundane but expected requirement now is access to television channels from around the world – including the Middle East – via satellite. Culinary delicacies from ethnic restaurants are commonly brought in so that families can spend evenings together enjoying food from their own countries. Avid readers of our own press will have noticed a certain interest in food produced by the Clinic in Michael Winner's regular column in the Sunday Times in 2007.

Although there was a maternity department at one time and inevitably some babies required specialist treatment (Figure 7.1), this service was discontinued in the late 1960s. Children were also admitted from the start. This practice did not continue, as the specialist care of children required special facilities that were not thought to be available in a hospital which primarily treated adults. Nowadays, children two years and older are routinely admitted for elective surgery – most commonly for ear, nose and throat conditions. The full range of paediatric and child care, however, is not appropriate except in a specialized hospital.

At the beginning, pressure on beds and finances was almost unknown. Patients were admitted a night or two before their operation and were given ample time to regain their strength and confidence before returning home.

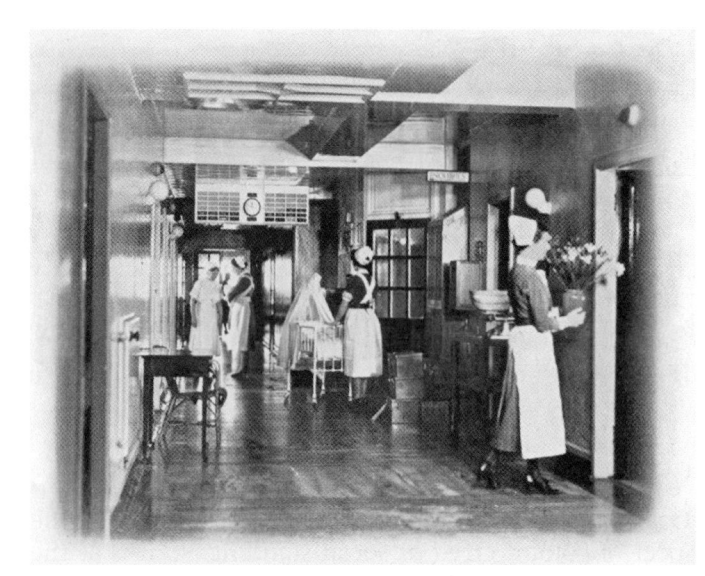

Figure 7.1
Maternity (seventh) floor.

It was not unusual for a husband to be admitted when his wife was awaiting delivery in the obstetric department, where beds (as in the rest of the Clinic) could be pre-booked. Such luxuries had to be pared in the face of a changing world of financial pressures, medical insurance and day surgery.

In order to be a patient at the Clinic, it was necessary to be under the care of a doctor on the British Medical Register who himself had admitting rights – this applied both to specialists and general practitioners. These had to be approved by a small house committee that included some of the prominent specialists themselves. They inevitably became powerful in regulating and protecting their own oligarchy. This, of course, was not unknown in the medical profession elsewhere in the country!

A former colleague of mine who spent a lifetime working in an NHS hospital – where patients can be made to feel grateful for gaining admission – chose private treatment for herself at the Clinic on four occasions. I solicited her testimony at random; she recalled only two minor deficiencies but was overwhelmingly impressed. She was met by friendly portering staff (Figure 7.2) and was then escorted via the Admissions Office to her room for the mandatory swab for methicillin-resistant *Staphylococcus aureus* (MRSA) and baseline readings of blood pressure and temperature. She was impressed by the daily cleaning inspection and the food, which was both good and hot. The nursing was excellent, with efficiency, kindness, continuity and compassion in the right proportions. Although not in any way well-to-do, she felt that the considerable insurance premiums had been an excellent investment. The testimony ended, 'I would not willingly go elsewhere – I rest my case'. I am sure the occasional 'disgruntled of Tunbridge Wells' exists; they are happily in the minority and, when identified, problems are investigated rigorously.

Patients

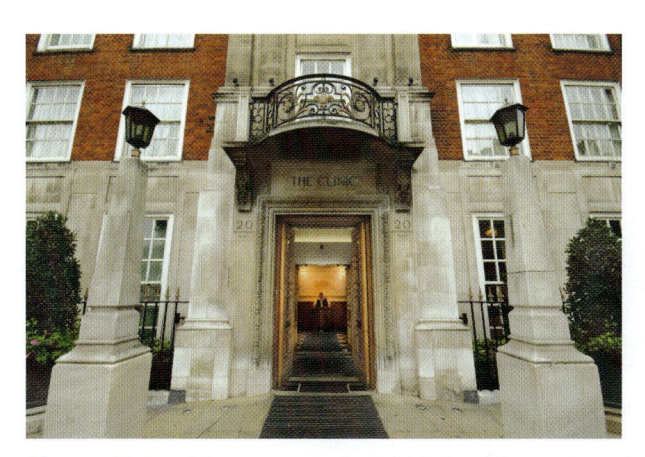

Figure 7.2 *The entrance by which inpatients are admitted – the reception desk that greets them can be seen.*

I myself arrived at the Clinic two or three years ago as an emergency by taxi in the early hours of the morning and was greeted with efficiency and caring concern. Entry is usually less precipitate, and most patients hopefully arrive in a more dignified way. There is a reassuring welcome at the front desk from someone who is not only knowledgeable but also able to project a calm confidence to anxious patients and relatives, who may not always be English. A ring of satellite offices look after admissions and accounts; the process of documentation required by the Clinic and the ever-growing requirements of insurance providers. When admission is complete, patients are conducted to their rooms. As well as being accompanied by a porter, mobile clothes hanging racks, usually only spotted in the best hotels, inevitably are available.

The administrative documentation required on admission is nowadays matched by the clinical documentation conducted by the nurses, which forms a new national ritual. Everyone is now aware of your disabilities, medical history and nickname – presumed to be essential requirements for programming your progress from infirmity to health.

The rather formal relationship that our own countrymen sometimes have towards their ailing relatives usually falls short of the support and devotion of many families from abroad. This has been a lesson for us all and may, to some extent, have prompted the Clinic to provide overnight beds for patients' relatives.

Patients' rooms (Figure 7.3) take on the character of those in temporary occupation. There is a whole spectrum of changes that are rung to suit the requirements of each patient. Only the extremes are really memorable. Tobacco smoke is now no longer in evidence, but the scent used by those from the Middle East lingers in rooms, even after the discharge of patients and the departure of bodyguards sitting outside their rooms. Alcohol is

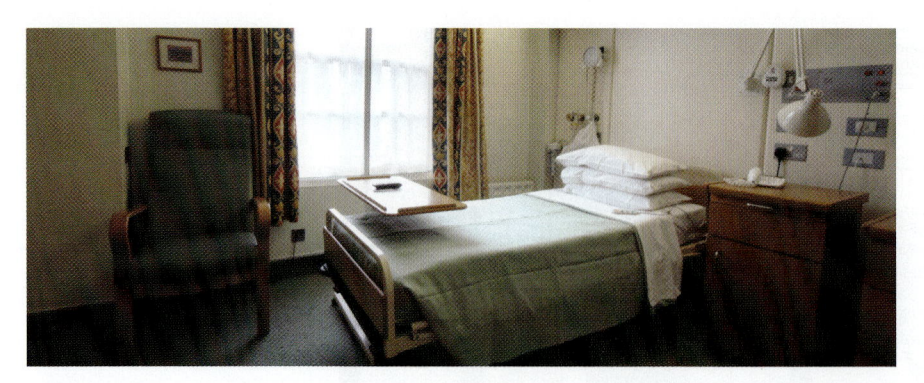

Figure 7.3 *A bedroom today.*

clearly therapeutic to some, and imported mezzes to others. Looking around the doors on an early morning visit confirms that we are all different – whether in sickness or in health. Some resist the call of dawn, while others devour newspapers avidly – occasionally wearing white gloves to avoid having newsprint on their hands. The radio headphones of the past are replaced by television screens, which can feature a number of programmes to satisfy almost every taste and culture.

All life is here – although births no longer take place intentionally. When a death occurs, the body is not now retained in the mortuary in the basement but despatched discreetly with an undertaker's supervision. On one occasion in my own experience, a wedding took place in a room – more for inheritance tax planning than as a result of an arrow from cupid's bow but nevertheless a wedding.

Great respect and affection usually is kindled between patients and nursing staff – and sometimes a fierce loyalty. On one occasion a sister was involved in a dispute with an uncontrollable patient. On seeing what was happening, another patient, who was not confined to his bed, leaped to assist crying, 'Man the telephone and make her tea!' Assaults in public hospitals are alas now more common and indeed more violent than this rare event at the Clinic.

8

The good, the bad and the ugly

Some of the patients who pass through the Clinic have been legends in their own lifetime from the worlds of politics, stage and screen, racing, literature and even royalty. Any notoriety and eccentricity that went before them is usually confirmed and developed during their time as patients. Some have been memorable merely by their grandeur in an era when royalty, national leaders and even mere politicians commanded greater awe and respect than today. In the past security was less in evidence, and the prying eyes of the media were both more restrained and more discreet. In due course, the patient base widened to include the wealthy, those with medical insurance (often as fringe benefits provided by employers) and, more recently, the international travelling circus of worried well and genuinely ill.

An early royal patient was Prince Arthur of Connaught, who, aged 88 years and with gastric trouble, was driven to the Clinic from his country house, Bagshot Park – now the home of the Earl and Countess of Wessex. Ever since his abdication as Edward VIII, the Duke of Windsor, and the Duchess, attracted the attention of the press. In 1959 and 1964, the Duchess spent time in the Clinic for what was described as 'facial surgery'. The Duke himself had surgery for a detached retina in 1965 (Figures 8.1 and 8.2). The president of India, Dr Radhakrishnan, had a cataract operation the same year. Princess Margaret underwent surgery on her face in 1980. Ex-Queen Aliyah of Iraq attracted attention as her son, the young King Faisal, was at Harrow. His cousin, King Hussain of Jordan, from time to time was a patient at the Clinic; when there, he kept his gold-plated revolver close at hand but entrusted it to the matron on the way to the operating theatre. When ex-King Umberto of Italy was a patient, a reporter from an Italian newspaper managed to gain entry dressed in a nurse's uniform. Happily his disguised camera was spotted, and the film destroyed. The deceptions of the press always provided a challenge to which the Clinic was usually able to rise, often successfully, as when the King of Siam required anonimity for a cataract operation.

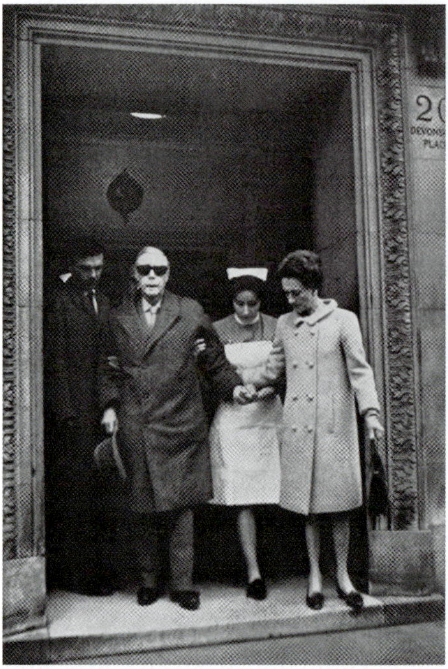

Figure 8.1 *The Duke and Duchess of Windsor leaving the Clinic in 1965 following his eye operation.*

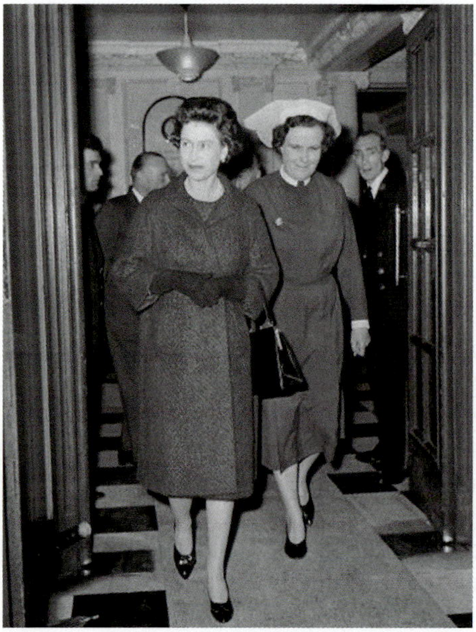

Figure 8.2 *HM The Queen, escorted by Matron Joan Lewis, leaving the Clinic after visiting her uncle, the Duke of Windsor. Reproduced with permission from PA photos.*

Affairs of State continued in patient's rooms from time to time during the Second World War and afterwards. The 'Council of Prices, Productivity and Income' met in the boardroom when Sir Harold Howitt was a patient. Ernest Bevin, as foreign secretary, required a scrambler telephone to be installed. Having previously been at the Clinic for the signing of the Cyprus treaty, Archbishop Makarios subsequently became a patient, and a generous-minded nurse described him as 'a sweet, kindly, strikingly handsome gentleman…and not at all like the Archbishop of Evil.' Anthony Eden, even before he was foreign secretary, always attracted attention – suave and well dressed, he sported a moustache (Figure 8.3). This was popular at the time but has become less fashionable – especially since the Lord Lucan scandal. In an issue of the *Yorkshire Evening News*, which featured the obituary of that early Clinic figure, Lord Moynihan, a headline read 'the talk of London – Mr Anthony Eden grows a beard.' One of his visits to the Clinic became much more than the talk of the town and attracted great international political attention. His continuing ill health almost certainly robbed him of the pre-

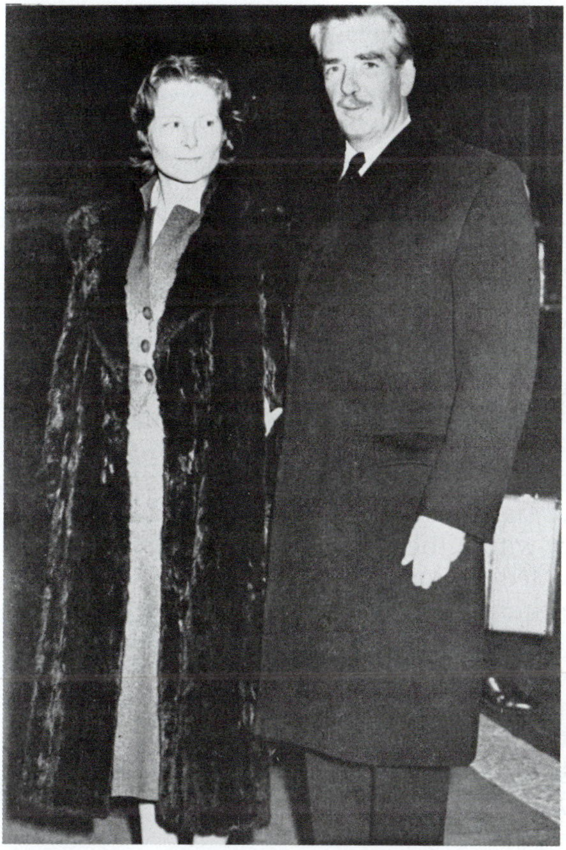

Figure 8.3 *Mr Anthony Eden (later Lord Avon), with his wife Clarissa, about to enter the Clinic before his gallbladder operation.*

miership. This was a sad hand to be dealt having survived the trenches in then First World War, in which two of his brothers had been killed.

The report of the original cholecystectomy operation that Eden underwent on 12 April 1953 did not record any problem; however, there was a complication with the free drainage of bile from the liver. The operation had been performed by Basil Hume, a general surgeon from St Bartholomew's Hospital. An explanation of the technical problem was never made public. Some years later, when being guided through a similar operation by Hume's surgical protégée (himself a consultant at the Clinic), I was instructed not to put traction on the common bile duct and cause a functional obstruction from 'tenting' of the duct. This causes an increase in pressure, and a ligature on the cystic duct could well be blown off – as was claimed in the case of Sir Anthony Eden. Ultimately, Eden went to the Lahey Clinic in Boston for the specialist skills of Dr Richard Cattell. This angered Winston Churchill, who stated that King George VI himself had been operated on at home – apocryphally on the kitchen table in Buckingham Palace. The latest authoritative account of Eden's operation, by the Right Honourable Lord (David) Owen, was published in the *Quarterly Journal of Medicine* on 1 June 2005 and can be found in Appendix 15.

Eden resigned in January 1957. The Suez invasion had not been a glorious chapter in British politics, with the intrigue of the Sevres protocol (which Eden denied publicly) preceding it. Thereafter, influence over the Middle East shifted from Europe to America, where it remains. I cannot help thinking that Eden's expressive turn of phrase about President Nasser taking over the canal being 'like a thumb on the windpipe' arose from his experience of a recent anaesthetic intubation!

Although Eden effectively walked off the British political stage in the Clinic, a politician from abroad, Seretse Khama, walked onto the stage on another occasion. He assumed responsibility for the future of Bechuanaland in the room of the dying chief Tshekedi. Some years earlier, Dr Chaim Weizman, president of the World Jewish Zionist Organization, underwent an operation for cataract that ultimately allowed him to assume the first presidency of Israel. His faith in the Clinic was confirmed when his wife Vera returned as a patient in 1966.

Over the years, the stars of stage, screen and radio have always found comfort, expertise and privacy within the Clinic's cocoon. Charlie Chaplin was operated on for an impacted wisdom tooth, with a much publicized demand from the US for the equivalent of £250,000 of tax arrears. Robert Morley was confined to the Clinic when rehearsals for the play the 'Staff Dance' with Barbara Lilley were taking place. Rehearsals were arranged in the mortuary in the basement. Some years later, Morley's mother-in-law, Gladys Cooper, was a patient. Richard Tauber, Joan Sutherland and Shirley Bassey entrusted themselves to the Clinic, as did Jacqueline du Pré, Nijinsky (star of the Diagalev Ballet), Nureyev and, more recently, Dame Alicia Markova.

The good, the bad and the ugly

The misfortunes of Elizabeth Taylor in 1961, however, led to more columns of newsprint than those of many, if not all, the other stars of stage and screen put together. Taylor was in London to make Cleopatra for 20th Century Fox. News of her pneumonia and tracheostomy jammed the switchboards of both the Clinic and the Dorchester Hotel, where she had been staying. The media vultures jockeyed for pole position for an exclusive story. In the end, the anaesthetist and the patient-triggered Barnett ventilator, which in those days was a rare piece of equipment, won the day. The whole world owned her infirmity, and those with money invested in the film had an anxious time. Despite the successful outcome and pictures of her leaving the Clinic (Figure 8.4), the satirical magazine *Private Eye* dubbed the Clinic a place where a person could die expensively rather than survive *gratis*. Happily, Elizabeth Taylor celebrated her 75th birthday this year – as did her brithday-twins, The London Clinic and the Regent's Park Open Air Theatre!

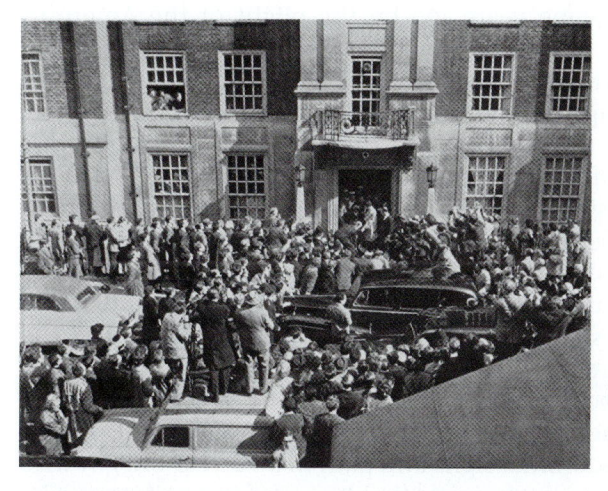

Figure 8.4 *Press interest in the discharge of Elizabeth Taylor in 1961.*

The young and memorably beautiful star Kay Kendal, remembered for her part in Genevieve, died in the Clinic of leukaemia when she was aged just 32 years; the world shared Rex Harrison's grief. Dickson Wright, a surgeon from St Mary's who worked at the Clinic, launched the Kay Kendal Memorial Fund, as he was treasurer of the Imperial Cancer Research Fund. He believed that this and other cancers could be cured by chemicals and therefore anticipated the great developments in chemotherapy that were to take place over the next 50 years. Despite this vision and foresight, Wright is perhaps better remembered for his remarkable surgical skills and wit as an after-dinner speaker.

The people who competed with themselves and nature in feats of speed and endurance often chose the Clinic when their bodies were harmed by their endeavours or their families needed care. Charles Lindbergh was surrounded by such notoriety after his solo flight across the Atlantic in 1927 and the subsequent kidnap (in March 1932) and killing of his son that he and his wife chose the peace and privacy of the Clinic for the birth of their second child soon afterwards. Fred Winter was to win the Grand National after a fracture of his leg was treated at the Clinic. Harry Carr, the Queen's jockey, had an injury treated at the Clinic in 1962. More recently Lester Piggott and Frankie Dettori have found themselves in the Clinic's parade ring.

Harold Larwood and Leslie Aimes were two of the early test cricketers to come to the Clinic. More recently, a fast bowler had to be brought from Lords for surgery: he had undergone stapled repair of a hernia with keyhole surgery before coming to this country. The staples had trapped the bowel, with disastrous consequences when he started his run up the wicket. When Robert Menzies, the former prime minister of Australia, visited England in 1968 to be installed as president of the Kent County Cricket Club, he had a stroke and was treated in the Clinic.

Many fishing stories circulate around the consultants at lunch and tea. These were supplemented some years ago by the plight of the American ambassador, Lewis Douglas, when he was fishing for salmon on the lower reaches of the Test. His host was Richard Fairey, head of the aviation firm that bore his name. Unhappily, the ambassador got a hook in his eye. Richard Fairey – previously a patient at the Clinic when both his legs were amputated after an encounter with a U-boat during the war – arranged for the ambassador to be transferred there. Among the many press reports of this event, I never remember reading whether the accident occurred when employing overhead rather than Spey casting or even the wind conditions. The accident probably would be analysed today by the Health and Safety Commission and guidelines issued about wearing spectacles to protect the riparian owners from the creeping legislative culture seen in society today – as the Clinic knows only too well.

Only after the Clinic had closed its maternity floor was a colleague of mine so confused by the abdominal signs and pain in a 12-year-old girl who was on a world tour with her grandparents that he called in a colleague. She was unexpectedly delivered of a healthy son. On another occasion, the matron had to deliver a baby in the lift in which she happened to be travelling with the mother. Fortunately at that time, it was still the tradition for the matron to wear a distinctive uniform, so the mother in labour had confidence in the rather unaccustomed midwife. The matron, distinguished by her uniform, did not have to be concerned about being accused of assault.

When Emil Savundranayagan was a patient in 1955 after he had been committed to Brixton Prison for fraud and forgery there was an application for a writ of *habeas corpus* to move him. However, the Home Office ordered that he should remain in the Clinic with a police constable at his bedside.

John Sainsbury, head of the provision merchants, sadly fell to his death from the fourth floor of the Clinic in 1956. Pain and depression played a part in this case, but many patients have left with publicity and photo calls. Nubar Gulbenkian, however, quietly tipped matron £5 on leaving.

9

Nursing

When it was necessary to think of engaging nurses as the Clinic opened, one of the leading clinicians was Lord Moynihan of Leeds. His judgement led to the appointment of Miss M Hebdon. Moynihan had worked all his life in Leeds, with regular sorties to London, where he was the most illustrious commercial traveller in surgery. When the Clinic was founded, he set up his stall there. It was not surprising that Miss Hebdon was translated from her position as matron at the Yorkshire Co-operative for Nurses and Nursing Homes Limited to the Clinic. Just how many nurses made the journey south is not known, but clearly she and Moynihan would have been a powerful magnet. Not all the floors were opened at once, so recruitment continued over the next few years.

At the time the Clinic went into receivership six months after opening, Miss Pinnell, who was assistant matron, became acting matron and, in turn, was succeeded by Jean Jacomb in 1938. Jacomb retired in 1949 and was followed by Miss Joan Lewis from St Mary's Hospital (see Appendix 3).

Medicine and surgery, it is said with much truth, can only be as good as the nursing staff. Nursing can only be as good as the matron. When opening a new hospital, there has to be a major recruitment of staff. The burden of responsibility for appointing the nurses inevitably falls on the matron. Having no training school, all the nurses had to be recruited widely – and in those days, as now, many of the best nurses over the years came not only from nursing schools within the UK but also from Eire. The net now is cast more widely across the globe. To choose a new workforce and engender both trust and discipline while developing the loyalty and morale so essential to good nursing care is still a demanding and vital task. The appointment of a formidable and experienced matron ensured that a reputation for excellent nursing quickly developed. This was maintained and fostered over the years by the provision of a residential nurses home and by meeting the needs of training and education that, in recent years, have become so essential.

Thirty years after the Clinic was founded, the sight of Sir Winston Churchill leaving the Devonshire Place entrance after visiting Anthony Eden with a confident matron immediately behind him projected to all the central role and importance of nursing (Figure 9.1). Although Sir Winston was merely visiting a patient, the matron was the most important member of the Clinic staff to accompany him when he left. None could fail to notice her almost regal appearance, which projected authority identifiable not only by her demeanour but also by her dress. This was immediately apparent to nurses, patients, the medical profession and the public. Such an image has now sadly submerged – but hopefully will surface again.

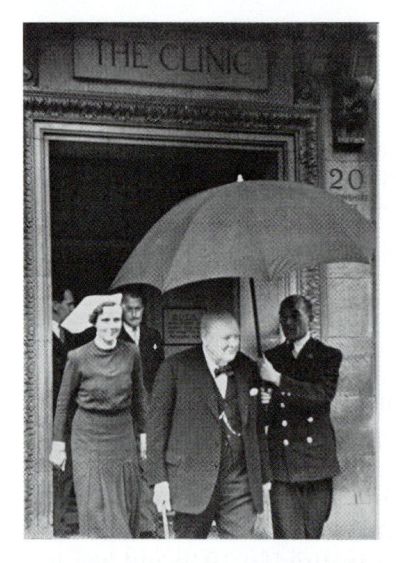

Figure 9.1 *Sir Winston Churchill escorted by Matron Joan Lewis.*

The nurses were initially accommodated in a hostel (Brendon House, Nottingham Place) from which they were able to walk to work. This was also possible from Osborne and Windsor Mews, 145 Harley Street, and 18 Devonshire Place, where nurses at one time were accommodated. A new home on the east side of Regents Park, Vernon House, was acquired by the Clinic as a nurses' home in the late 1950s (Figure 9.2). This had 100 single rooms and a dining area. A bus originally carried the day shift to work, returning with the night shift. After 40 years, the accommodation required for nurses was changing. Three of the terrace houses were converted back to large private dwellings and sold, and the proceeds used to refurbish the rest as individual studio flats. This redevelopment was opened by Lady Hartington (now the Duchess of Devonshire) in July 1999.

Some of the original uniforms can be seen illustrated on page 15, 52 and 64. Sisters had long sleeves and fly-away caps, and nurses short sleeves and stiff white aprons with crossover straps behind (Figure 7.1). The ritual of when and where to change aprons and white cuffs became firmly established in

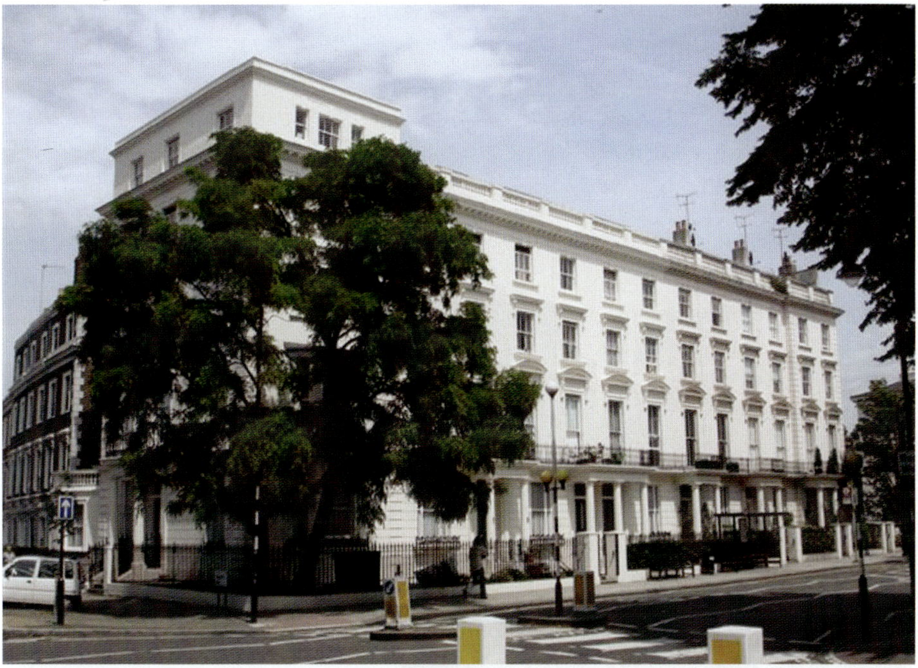

Nursing 63

Figure 9.2 *Vernon House nurses' hostel in Regents Park.*

nursing practice in this country. This undoubtedly had a place in hygiene, which started to be lost when the cost of a labour-intensive laundry service became an issue. One can but speculate how this (as well as the inappropriate use of antibiotics) contributed to the growing problem of cross-infection and super bugs that we see today.

This change in culture occurred not merely at the Clinic but universally across the whole country. In addition to the length of sleeves and the wearing of aprons, seniority was also colour-coded. Sisters were in green (Figure 9.4), charge nurses in blue with red belts and the most junior nurses in cobalt blue with navy belts. The original dresses were designed and tailored by a fashionable designer of the time, Boyd Cooper; the firm, like the Clinic, is still in business. Later, the traditional dresses and aprons were changed to all-white uniforms with coloured trims, and a choice of trousers as an alternative to dresses.

The various agency nurses who may be required to support the permanent staff introduce some variety, but they are identified only with certainty by name-badges with the logo of their nursing agency. Patients and doctors peer at their labels of origin in the way that visitors peer at the names of plants in the hot-houses at Kew. Pretty hairstyles may give individuals self-confidence, but to some the old uniformity of head-dresses and

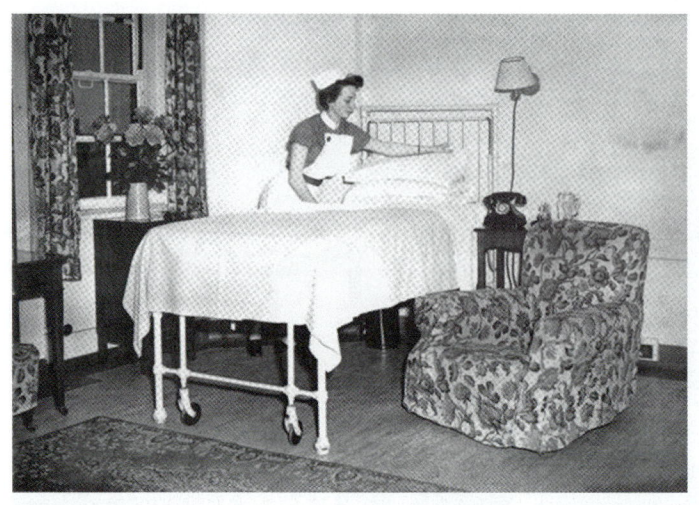

Figure 9.3 *Original nurses uniform (compare with sisters uniform in Figure 2.5).*

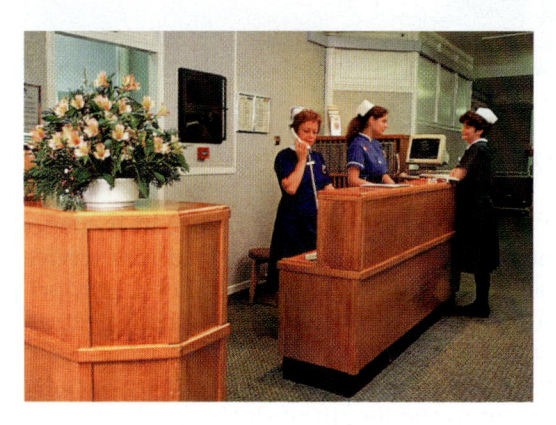

Figure 9.4 *Anne Ducey, Martine McDowell, Marie Carton (from left to right), seen wearing their uniforms and caps – photograph taken in the early 1990s.*

aprons generated pride and increased the corporate identity. This may even have helped combat cross-infection. It seems remarkable that headgear is required by those preparing food in the kitchens but not by nursing staff who may be changing dressings in the ward. Work on the nasal carriage of staphylococci by bacteriologists such as Professor Reginald Shooter and Professor Francis O'Grady at St Bartholomew's Hospital in the 1960s and resulting cross-infection in the wards seems to have sunk into temporary obscurity. Thankfully, dispensers of bactericidal solutions have recently been reintroduced outside the rooms of particularly vulnerable patients in the Clinic.

By the time Jean Jacomb succeeded as matron in 1938, the Clinic was well established and stable. Even more than now, the character and presence of the matron was important in maintaining the efficiency and discipline of any hospital. Standards can be maintained by discipline, example or fear. Usually, there is a subtle and often unconscious fusion of all three. Jean Jacomb's tenure was said to be a period of happiness, with a gentle but firm hand guiding the tiller. When she retired in 1949, her assistant, Joan Lewis, took up the reins. Having trained at St Mary's Hospital, she was comfortably surrounded by many consultants from her own teaching hospital. She worked at Park Prewett Mental Hospital in Basingstoke during the war and initially joined the Clinic as night sister before becoming assistant matron.

Sylvia Dutton, who followed as matron from 1967 to 1979, exercised command over the Clinic with traditional discipline but was approachable to all and had an enviable blend of understanding, discipline and compassion in her dealings with patients, nurses and consultants (Figure 9.5). She recognized that times were beginning to change and that the Clinic should also change and develop. An example of this was the help she gave in establishing the endoscopy unit. Perhaps it was not insignificant that Dr Basil Morson, the internationally acclaimed colorectal pathologist from St Mark's Hospital, was now working in the pathology department. He brought the benefit of his wisdom to this department at the Clinic and became a friend of the matron. They subsequently married. Sylvia Dutton's contribution to private nursing was recognized when she became a Member of the Order of the British Empire (MBE).

Laura Henderson, who was matron from 1979 to 1984, had served under Sylvia Dutton and continued to maintain traditional standards in the face of all the changes that were overtaking the profession (Figure 9.6). She was full of ideas for the benefit of the Clinic and nurses, but many of them were far ahead of their time and therefore were not implemented.

Henderson's place was, in turn, taken by her deputy, Betty Boden (Figure 9.7), who was matron from 1984 to 2003 and whose career at the Clinic started as a staff nurse in 1969. Within a year, she became a sister and, after being a departmental head, she became deputy matron in 1980. Her years as matron were a period of transition, involving changes that ranged from new technology to employment law and from budgets to the Care

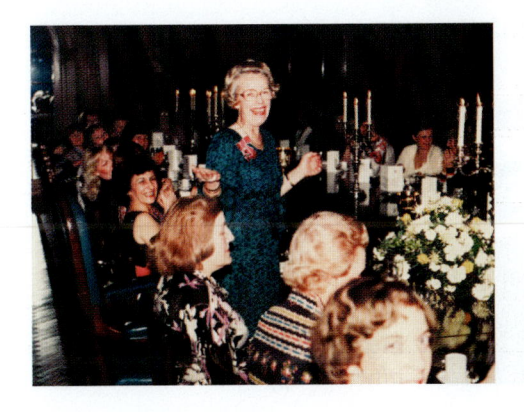

Figure 9.5 *Sylvia Dutton at her retirement party.*

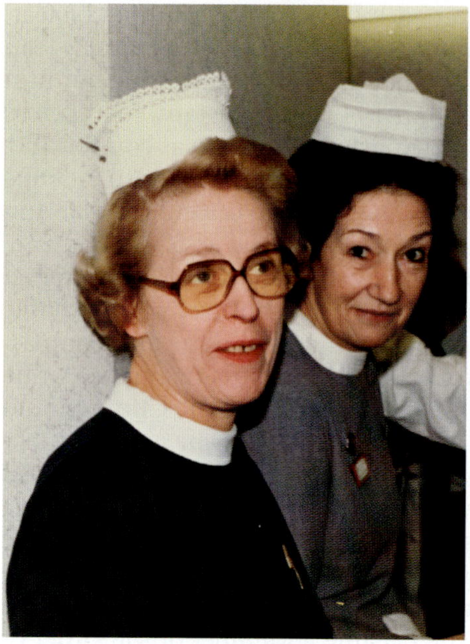

Figure 9.6 *Sylvia Dutton (foreground) and her successor Laura Henderson.*

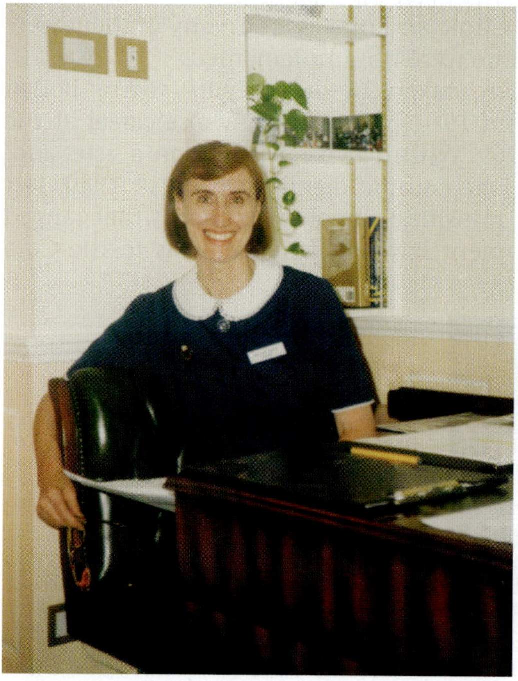

Figure 9.7 *Betty Boden shortly after her appointment as matron.*

Standards Commission. All the time the vagaries of the insurance companies, as well as the new competitive market, had to be kept in view. These challenges were faced successfully, with a cauldron of care and efficient organization that led to the King's Fund's award to the Clinic in 1999.

Historically, matrons had lived on the premises, but, in the search for space, their flat initially became the health screening unit and later the MRI unit. There is still residential accommodation for the on-call medical officers, however, and the chairman has a flat for his use when in London. Accommodation in one or other of the properties in Harley Street leased by the Clinic is provided for on-call staff from the theatre, pharmacy and pathology department.

The specialization that developed meant that nursing floors needed to have specific skills. Orthopaedics was located on the sixth floor, in close proximity to the hydrotherapy pool. Gynaecology and breast care were sited on the fifth floor. The diminishing specialty of general surgery shared the fourth floor with the minimally invasive treatment unit (MITU) at the east end, while colorectal and progressive care occupied the third floor. The ever-increasing empire of oncology could not be contained on one floor, so it spread from the second to the first floor, with ear, nose and throat (ENT) and ophthalmology fitted in between. The old boardroom has even yielded to the pressure for clinical space, but the chief executive, like King Canute, bravely holds onto his office – where, in fact, he is best placed to keep his finger on the administrative pulse.

All of these changes underlined the need for the continuing education of nurses through their professional life. It was during Betty Boden's time that the nurse education department was set up in 145 Harley Street in 1980 and entrusted to Anna Steven, a sister at the Clinic. The concept of the 'nursing process' was introduced on all nursing floors. Being in the vanguard of this process, the Clinic was approached by St Bartholomew's Hospital's nursing education department to take student nurses on placement. This was an early example of co-operation between the NHS and the private sector. There are now placements for 30 nursing, 20 radiology and six physiotherapy students linked with the City of London University.

A reference library was started, and internal lectures and courses introduced. Some of these were given by consultants who worked at the Clinic. Nurses also started to specialize and take the Nursing Board's qualifications in their specialist area. This enabled a wide range of specialities, including stoma care, outreach into the community, infection control, endocrinology, dialysis, oncology and breast care to be accommodated. Nurses became responsible for individual patients during their entire admission. An appraisal system was implemented. Although this seemed very novel, and indeed now applies to consultants, a similar requirement was actually in place in the Arab hospitals in Damascus in the early eighth century!

The educational programme enabled nurses to convert from enrolled to registered nurses. Other staff were also taken under the wing of the nursing education department. Ultimately, the responsibility for education was formally taken into the human resources (HR) department led by Gillian Irvine. Other services, such as those provided by Cancerbackup and Macmillan Nurses, are now grafted onto the specialist nursing skills. There are also counselling services for a number of conditions including breast disease, liver disease and gynaecology. Among all this education and specialization, sight was not lost of the fact that nurses minister to patients' needs 24 hours a day.

After Betty Boden retired (Figure 9.8), Amanda Hallums – who had never worked in the Clinic – was brought in from Basildon and Thurrock University Hospitals NHS Trust, where she was director of nursing, to be matron (Figure 9.9). She had trained at the Royal London Hospital, Whitechapel, where she became a ward sister, before moving to Whipps Cross Hospital. Her task will be to blend the best from tradition with the demands of the present day – surely a challenging task. Recruitment and retention of nursing staff, training and skill–mix will inevitably be top of her personal agenda. To maintain the present ratio of 1:4 nurses per patient will be an important task for her.

No account of nursing would be complete without mention of matron's office, which may be regarded as a command centre, bunker, Cabinet war room and mission control all in one. This conjures up a picture ranging from a map table with service leaders planning the deployment of forces,

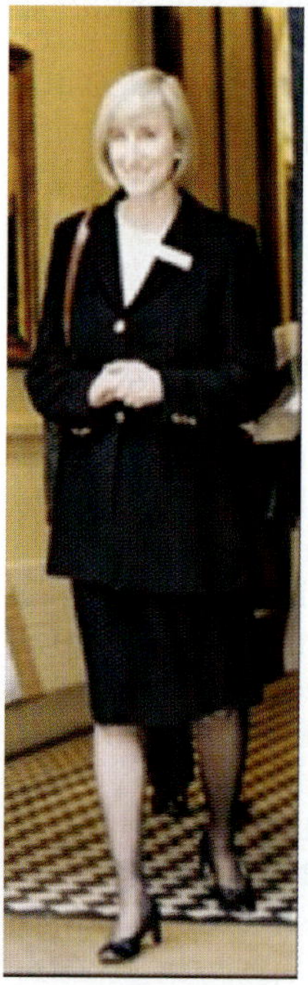

Figure 9.8 *Betty Boden leaving 145 Harley Street shortly before her retirement.*

Nursing

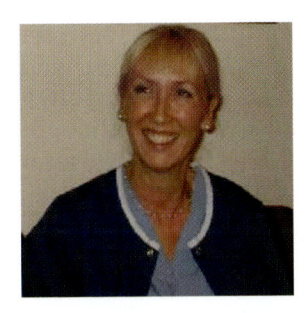

Figure 9.9 *Amanda Hallums.*

the German High Command in the dark days of 1940 and Churchill planning allied strategy. In keeping with modern times, it could also be likened to mission control at the National Aeronautics and Space Administration (NASA). All are embodied in matron's office. By day, admissions and bookings (patient liaison) have separate offices, but matron's office is their understudy at night and, indeed, sets the stage over every 24 hours. Although some day nurses in most hospitals undertake night shifts, a special cohort of dedicated nurses undertake the night watch at the Clinic – sometimes for many years, such as Marjorie Corner, who was night superintendent. Matron's office controls the chorus of nurses and soloists from each movement or act of an endless clinical 'Ring Cycle' reminiscent of Wagner. It also needs a proscriptive and ruthless Teutonic efficiency to make everything run to the patients' advantage. Within the office's remit are all those other aspects of managing people and communities – discipline, training and off-duty that achieve cohesion like super-glue. Moreover, the office is placed strategically by the main entrance, so that matron knows exactly who is coming and going, even monitoring traffic wardens through the window.

Despite all their care, however, occasional problems slip through their net. In 1976, a disgruntled agency nurse, Miss Kay Simon, developed a grudge against private medicine. She threatened that the Clinic would be blown up unless money was left at Euston Station. This threat to the placid progress of life at the Clinic was circumvented by the police.

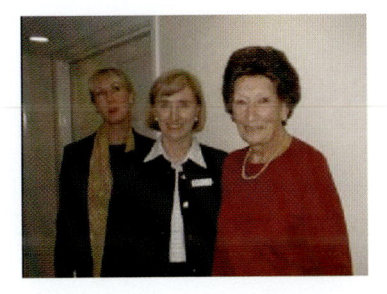

Figure 9.10 *A pride of matrons – Amanda Hallums, Betty Boden and Laura Henderson (from left to right).*

Although there is no Clinic chaplaincy or non-denominational room for prayer, meditation and counselling, matron's office holds lists of those who can be called on to minister to families of the bereaved. The Clinic originally had a mortuary and chapel in the basement, but these were thought to be a dispensable luxury that only served limited use in a somewhat secular age – and the space was required for essential clinical developments.

10

Physiotherapy, phlebotomists and interpreters

Physiotherapy

In the 1950s, Frank Anyan was given the task of developing a physiotherapy department. The first home was in an old operating theatre on the seventh floor. As the dependence on physiotherapy in many aspects of clinical care grew, four rooms were taken over on the first floor in 1970, and the department grew with the appointment of Patricia George. After a move to the ground floor of 18 Devonshire Place in 1973, a final home was found on the sixth floor of 147 Harley Street, with a custom-built gym (Figure 10.1), hydrotherapy pool and several individual treatment rooms with various modalities of treatment, such as ultrasound. These were visited by the Prince of Wales in 1989 (Appendix 9).

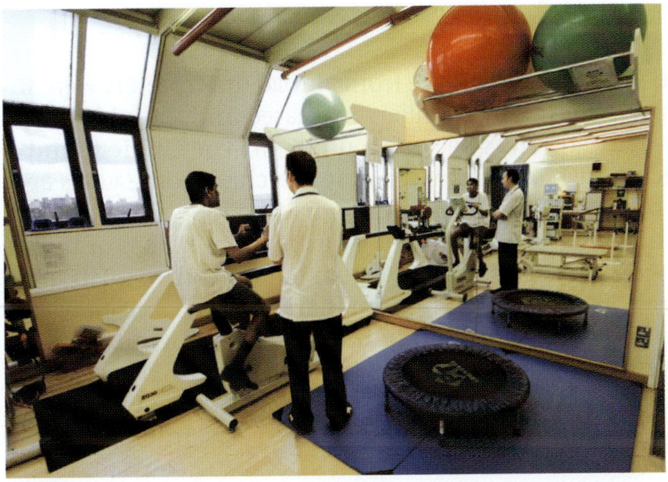

Figure 10.1
Physiotherapy department's gymnasium on the sixth floor.

Both inpatients and outpatients are treated. If inpatients are unable to visit the department, itinerant disciplinarians in the form of physiotherapists descend after the routine of breakfast, bed making and phlebotomy. They have disarming smiles that mask the physical attributes of 'Miss Joan Hunter Dunn' of blessed Betjeman memory and coax flagging chests and limbs into action.

Back in the department, as the day progresses, there is a steady stream of sports injuries and a procession of old contemptibles (getting younger all the time) who have had their hips replaced. As they float in the hydrotherapy pool, they exercise their new joints and fantasize about being weightless spacemen with mission control bringing them back to earth and returning them to their previous life and pleasures. Happily this is now often the case.

In both inpatients and outpatients, the role of physiotherapy in preventing postoperative chest infections and deep vein thrombosis, and also in aiding recovery after strokes and orthopaedic and soft tissue surgery cannot be overestimated.

Phlebotomists

Like vultures circling from the Towers of Silence in India, phlebotomists visit the nursing floors, descending here and there with trays of sample tubes, syringes and request forms – returning to the laboratory with their samples. The results can now be obtained online from automatic analysers, without the frustrations of misfiled results and telephone calls. One other thing has changed in recent years – the phlebotomists have to take rigorous precautions against HIV/AIDS and other infections by using disposable gloves. The clinical scene is ever growing in complexity.

Interpreters

When prominent patients started to arrive from abroad, interpreters were included in their retinue. When their numbers increased and individuals began to arrive, however, interpreters became a problem. The Clinic found it difficult to communicate with a wealthy Chinese merchant some years ago, and an appeal was made for Chinese-speaking nurses to look after him and interpret. The need thereafter was often met by using the services of nurses or cleaners from abroad – most commonly Greek, Italian and Spanish nurses and more recently those from the Philippines and Eastern Europe.

The influx of Arab patients – for not all of them brought their own interpreters – led to a full time Arab interpreter being engaged. Pierre Maher Francis-Saati, Hoda Buckley and Rania Kaldos have served the Clinic with great sensitivity, understanding and courtesy over the years, interpreting for patients from many countries, including Greece.

11
Catering

Special diets were a feature of the Clinic from the beginning, and the advanced catering equipment has previously been listed in an earlier chapter. As the medical world changes its views about cholesterol, high fibre and salt, the kitchen staff have to play an attentive role of 'follow my leader', with a dietician walking the floors co-ordinating the clinical requirements and personal fads. When a diabetic patient suggested the need for diabetic desserts one Thursday evening, the kitchen responded, and diabetic puddings appeared on the menu by Tuesday (despite Monday being a bank holiday)!

From the beginning, each floor had a kitchen pantry where the trolleys from the main kitchen in the basement (Figure 11.1) could be parked and

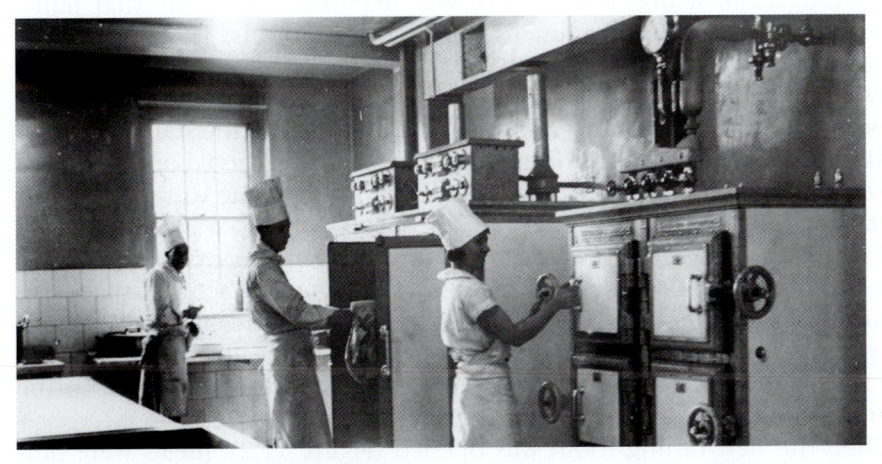

Figure 11.1   *The original kitchen.*

from which meals could be served. Institutional, particularly hospital, food always attracts a certain amount of ridicule. However, on the whole, the meals are hot, varied and nutritious. Certainly a lot of effort and planning has always gone into the patients' meals. When the kitchens are allowed to show off for a retirement party and at Christmas, exceptional and memorable fare is provided with great enthusiasm and pride. It is no mean task to produce several hundred meals with individual requirements all through the year and on public holidays. Over the years, this challenge has attracted a variety of chefs with varied backgrounds, including the Royal Yacht.

The attention paid to the original kitchens and the importance of food and special diets was to some extent eclipsed over the years by costs, solvency and the demands of clinical services. Those who are convalescent, however – like the army – march on their stomachs, and general well-being and good food (and even the Clinic's cellar!) cannot be neglected.

Some 30 years after the opening, it was necessary to look formally at the catering arrangements. The system introduced in the thirties had undergone little alteration. The initiative for this critical look at catering was put in place by Gilbert Rees. One of the issues was that the provision of food on the ward was very labour intensive – even taking the nurses and sisters away from clinical duties and, worse still, the visiting consultants.

The system of the nurses taking a menu to each patient, collating the information and contacting the kitchen was not an efficient use of their time. Compounding this were the decibels issuing from the service area on the wards. When the clatter of plates and the tannoy used to communicate with the service area was added, the system was clearly unsatisfactory. The stately progress of the trolleys from the kitchens was so slow that when the cortège arrived on the nursing floor the food was only tepid. A-la-carte imagination was not stretched and did not walk hand-in-hand with culinary innovation. A hospital messiah was required in the way that Jamie Oliver was later to seize the limelight with school meals. There was, however, no messiah but a working party which started a recruitment drive. Links were established with local catering colleges with the offer of resident accommodation to junior catering staff. Restructuring of the staff took place so that there was a *chef de partie* and *commis chef*. Food served on trays, centralized washing up and two new lifts almost brought the Clinic into consideration for Michelin stars.

Along with these changes, the staff dining arrangements were altered. This was necessary for all sorts of reasons, including the fact that space was required to accommodate the move of operating theatres from the eighth floor to the basement. The existing dining rooms that were exclusive to sisters, nurses and doctors were relocated to the area previously used for sitting rooms for nursing staff and sisters.

When the new dining room was opened (Figure 11.2), meals were purchased in a cook–chill form and warmed up in the dining room. Regrettable as this in some ways seemed to be, it did allow the best use of available

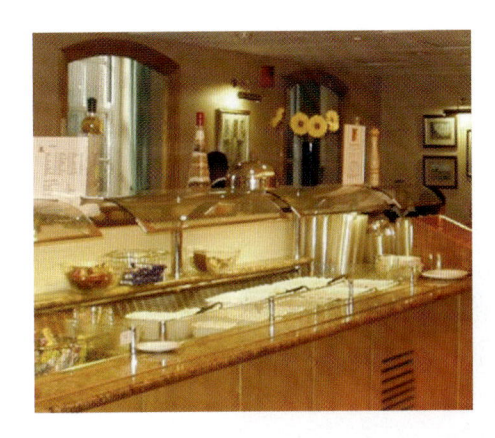

Figure 11.2 *Staff dining room today.*

space. Staff were free to serve the needs of the patients, and this approach also enabled the greatly increased numbers of nurses, administrative staff and doctors to be fed on site. The Clinic at this time entered the cashless swipe-card era, which made many realize that smart cards were indeed smarter and quicker than many had previously acknowledged.

More recently, it has proved possible for the Clinic kitchens to provide food for the staff dining room rather than purchasing it in cook–chill form (Figure 11.3). This provides a greater variety and better quality of food, meeting the needs of vegetarians and those who like a baguette on the hoof. The kitchens are able to produce some 200 meals for the staff dining room at lunch (Figure 11.4), in addition to the regular and occasional demands of the patients. This sometimes includes an individually cooked salmon that has to be moist, tender and cooked and borne to the patient personally by the chef, together with a bottle of champagne traditionally wrapped in a freshly laundered linen towel! The kitchen is also required to provide food for the night staff and patients who may feel they are suffering from night starvation. This is indeed sometimes the case if they have been nil-by-mouth because of a clinical procedure.

This catering revolution did not, however, sweep away the coffee and light meals facility for patients and relatives, which is known as 'The Terrace' and is located on the fifth floor (Figure 13.4). This continuing haven of peace and traditional service is enjoyed and appreciated by anxious relatives and friends. When the Clinic is redeveloped internally, space will be allocated to meet this requirement. In order to address any complaints, a quality assurance programme, in which problems are identified and changes monitored over the succeeding months, is now built in to the catering department. For those who wish to be familiar with the way hotel services have to be organized, it is mandatory in the Clinic for supervisors to have a level III National Vocational Qualification (NVQ). They earn a bonus on successful completion and those in the kitchen have to demonstrate their

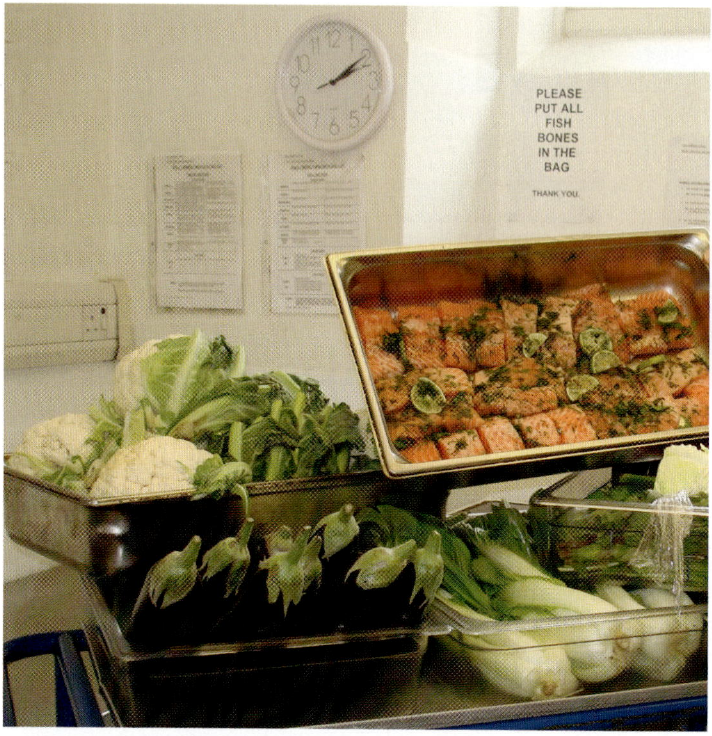

Figure 11.3 *Raw ingredients.*

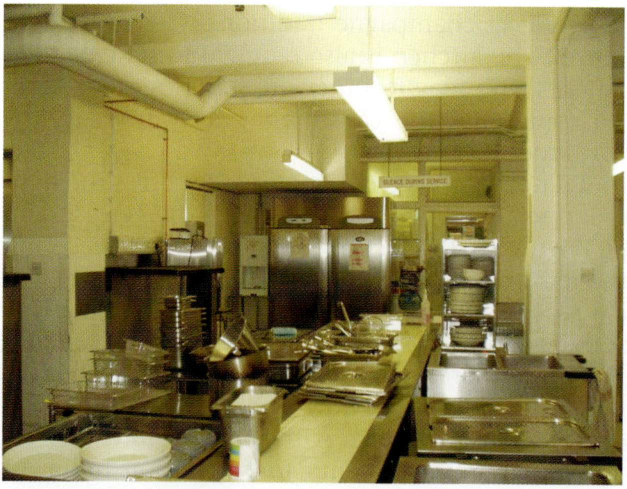

Figure 11.4 *Kitchen today.*

competence by achieving a level II NVQ. The rigid training and supervision that catering demands means that those with these qualifications have proved themselves and often move on within the Clinic to other positions, leading to a good overall retention of staff. This is particularly attractive to the new influx of staff from Eastern Europe who are highly motivated and wish to achieve their full potential.

12

Trace elements – clinical essentials

Switchboard

The best of relationships usually exists between the switchboard and the doctors. From the start of their careers, doctors have accepted the importance of this nerve centre for communications. This was especially so before the era of bleeps, when emergencies, cover, off-duty and advice about everything including taxis and pubs was channelled through the switchboard. It was always good to put a face to a voice and exchange a few words of greeting if the switchboard was by the hospital entrance when the emergency bleep was collected at the start of a spell on duty. At one time this was the case at the Clinic, but now the switchboard and operators are hidden in the basement and do not occupy prime space in the front hall. They fulfil their vital function and, in addition, continue to act as a cross between a chat-room and doctors-reunited. Their importance is not just for doctors but for patients, relatives and the ever-increasing host of administrators. The switchboard operators need special skills and understanding of the fact that everyone who telephones believes they are the only important caller. I am sure that they would need but minimal training to become Samaritans!

Three staff and a supervisor are on switchboard duty between the hours of 8 am and 10 pm and take up to 3,000 incoming calls a day. These are of varying complexity and often make great demands on tact and initiative. Calls at night are received by the reception desk at Devonshire Place. Among the important aspects of the job are the responsibilities for calls regarding cardiac arrests, security and fire alarms.

Porters, receptionists and couriers

The porters, receptionists and couriers provide a visible interface between the Clinic and the outside world. Trained to greet, help, respond and deliver everything from x-rays to flowers and newspapers, they provide a welcoming and efficient service and are full of friendly confidence (Figure 12.1). The jargon with which such essential skills are described today by those behind the scenes of the NVQs is 'customer facing' – an ugly phrase indeed.

In addition to providing a service for the Clinic and its satellites, they run errands and convey reports and specimens to and from the consulting rooms of specialists situated in Harley Street and the neighbouring streets.

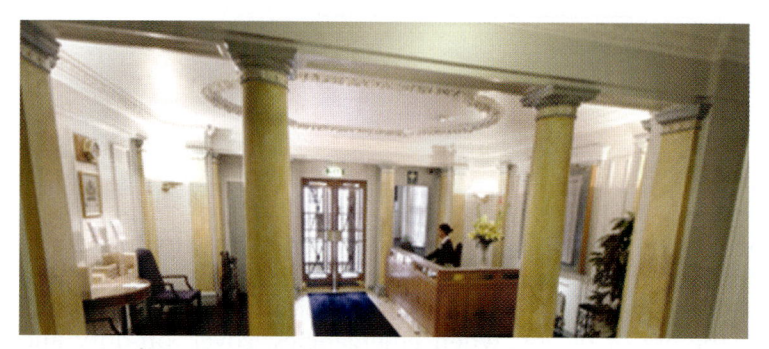

Figure 12.1 Reception, 149 Harley Street.

Housekeeping

One of the aspects of the staff that is immediately obvious, apart from their thorough and well-regimented efficiency, is what a happy team they form. This is evident from the moment one enters a lift with two or three going on duty or from a chance meeting in a corridor when wheeling a trolley of requisites as they undertake their various duties, which range from the pleasant to the unpleasant; all of which are undertaken with equal good humour. Their supervisors seem to be notably good communicators despite language barriers and are sympathetic task masters. They ensure a clean environment that must help to reduce hospital infections. They also provide Vernon House with caretakers and supervise the general day-to-day running.

Some necessarily have important and specialist roles. As you would expect in a hospital, the responsibility for collecting clinical waste and used needles is entrusted to a special porter. The transfer of beds and soiled linen also has to be undertaken with care and monitored.

A seamstress oversees the uniforms, including the labelling, the regular cleaning and any repair, all of which is not only important for cleanliness but necessary to maintain a smart corporate image.

Maintenance

Attending to the countless jobs that are always present in a large and busy organization – whether replacing light bulbs or television sets, mending doors and locks or attending to the plumbing – is the maintenance team. They enjoy a variety of tasks that are made more pleasant by meeting the patients and having the satisfaction of sharing in the immediate pleasure and gratitude when a problem is solved.

Purchasing and stores

Everything from paper to soap, crockery to linen and equipment to drugs has to be purchased, stored and distributed. The responsibility for this rests on the broad shoulders of the stores and purchasing department under Mike Sims. The power of bulk buying and repeat orders is a hand that has to be skilfully played: the market-place is ruthless and it now requires a very experienced team that has budgetary constraints.

The purchasing and stores department originally formed part of the pharmacy department at the Clinic and functioned as a small offshoot for the delivery of small consumable items. Over the last 17 years, the role and tempo of work has increased so dramatically that the purchasing department, as it is now known, functions as a totally independent unit from the pharmacy. Although it is one of the smaller departments, it has a vast pivotal and wide-reaching role, providing services to every department – clinical and non-clinical – in the central Clinic, its outreach departments at Park Square and 5 Devonshire Place and its satellites along Harley Street. It is responsible for the sourcing, purchasing and distribution of clinical and non-clinical equipment and consumables for all departments, and its philosophy is 'The right products, of the right quality, at the right time and at the right price'.

The team of eight comprises a purchasing manager, stores manager, purchasing assistant and five storekeeping staff. The need for close teamwork is absolute in order to manage and process the supply chain throughout the hospital daily to a very tight programme as supply requirements usually exceed the storage ability. To compensate for this necessitates the use of a 'just-in-time' system. There is a need to place orders with main distributors on one day and for the goods to arrive the next. The team receive, check and deliver most items to departments before or just after midday. This system has to be closely managed and monitored, as any delays in the daily process can have a knock-on effect that could hamper the operational efficiency of departments, particularly those with an acute service role. When selecting new suppliers, their ability to meet next-day supply is a major consideration.

The purchase of capital equipment usually involves high expenditure, particularly with scanners for computed tomography (CT) and Magnetic

Resonance Imaging (MRI) and more recently the da Vinci robotic surgical system. Such purchases are dealt with in a different manner from the approach taken by most large group organizations such as the NHS. Generally, they have a specific department that operates outside the hospitals' purchasing departments with the sole role of sourcing, contracting and negotiating for capital items. Within the Clinic, the purchasing department has a large input into capital purchases by working independently with the end specialist user to select the right equipment and by conducting checks on the supplier and manufacturer to ensure the equipment poses no risks in the Clinic.

Despite its small size, the purchasing department plays a diverse and vital role in maintaining a supply chain to most departments – including housekeeping and theatres, who also undertake some of their own purchasing. It has been developed in recent years under the leadership of Mike Sims.

13

The front line – 149 Harley Street

Consultants' offices – known as 'rooms' – have been housed in 149 Harley Street since the Clinic was opened (Figure 13.1). The building that previously occupied some of the site had been the home of John Kenyon, the poet and philanthropist, who spent his life in travel, dilettantism and dispensing charity – including helping Robert and Elizabeth

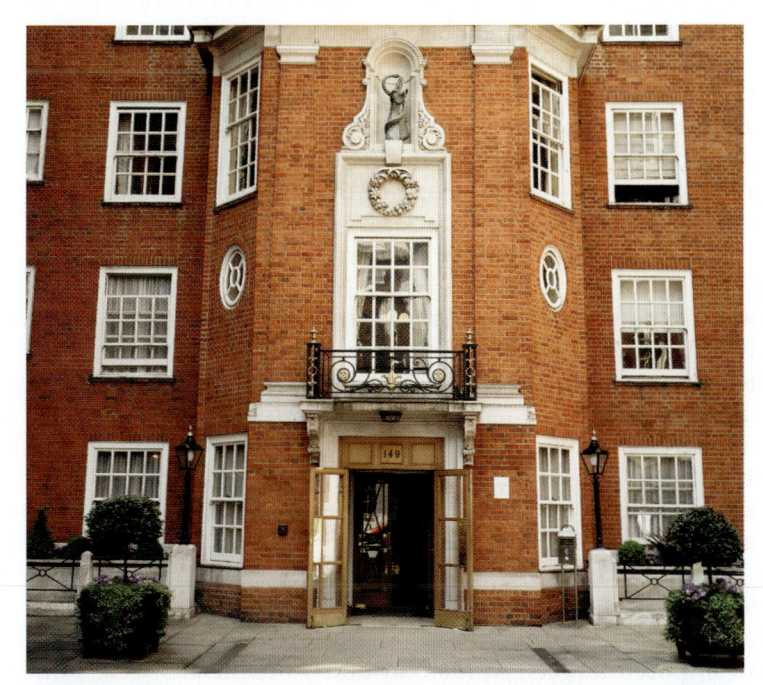

Figure 13.1 *Courtyard entrance of 149 Harley Street today.*

Browning, to whom he was a true friend. In 1848, his former home was acquired by Sir James Kay-Shuttleworth (1804–77), who was sometimes called 'the founder of English popular education'. By 1861, number 149 was occupied by Henry Methold, serjeant-at-law, who commuted each day to his legal chambers in Chancery Lane.

In 1879, the property passed into medical use when the physician, James Burnett, lived there. He was followed in the 1880s by Dame Mary Ann Dacomb Scharlieb (1845–1903), the gynaecological surgeon. Mary Ann's mother had died five days after her birth and because of the influence of an enlightened stepmother she received an excellent education. It is said that she was fond of riding but never joined in games and disliked dances and parties. In 1865, she met her future husband, William Mason Scharlieb of Madras, who was in England reading for the bar. From her husband's clients and clerks, she learned of the sufferings of the Hindu and Mohammedan women and determined to qualify as a doctor in order to help them. Against tremendous opposition, she and three other women qualified at the Madras Medical School in 1877. After a period abroad, and having founded the Royal Victoria Hospital for Caste and Gosha women at Madras, her health failed and she returned once more to London – and ultimately to 149 Harley Street. She became senior surgeon at the new hospital for woman (afterwards known as the Elizabeth Garrett Anderson Hospital). Since the reconstruction of 149 Harley Street when the Clinic was built in 1929, many distinguished practitioners have been happy to practice at this famous address.

From the start, the Clinic was served by an inner circle of favoured and usually nationally and internationally distinguished consultants. There was always a cross-section of specialists from the various disciplines. This inevitably became like a club – perhaps one of the most desirable medical clubs in the country. The waiting list for rooms in 149 was handwritten in the back of the house governor's minute book and inspected from time to time at the end of medical committees. Blackballing resulted in the equivalent of the editorial blue pencil being drawn through the name of those thought to be unacceptable. As well as clinical excellence, the influences of freemasonry, rugby and teaching hospitals were never far away. At the time, however, it worked and served the patients and the Clinic well.

As patients and beds had to be underpinned by developments in diagnosis and care, which were becoming ever more complicated, much was to change in this world of elegance and privilege. These clinical developments were extensive and had to be fed by a steady flow of patients in order to balance the books. The old stately progress through the clinical hoops of previous years became a roller coaster dictated by the pressures of patient demand as well as the insurance companies and ultimately the present culture of audit and imposed targets. At first, around 30 clinicians were sufficient to fill the beds and provide a complete range of specialities. This was all to change.

The front line – 149 Harley Street

Initially the waiting list for consulting rooms was many years – even if your face and skills seemed to fit. Others who were not in number 149 and some trusted and prominent general practitioners also brought patients to the Clinic and kept the beds fully occupied. With the easing of the Howard de Walden policy on licences, it was possible, officially, to have multiple licences to accommodate more consultants in rooms on a sessional basis. This, of course, had always been practised to some extent when junior consultants helped look after the patients of their seniors and in return were allowed to have some patients in their own right. Nowadays, some 140 specialists practise from the Clinic's consulting rooms and maintain bed occupancy (Figure 13.2). The consultants also have a much broader international origin than was the case 20 years ago.

The Victorian drawing-room culture of consultations is now disappearing. It had been a world of privilege for a few, and undoubtedly the desirable working conditions and rewards lured consultants, on occasions, from their responsibilities with the NHS. This was justified by the claim that their absence allowed the juniors at their NHS hospitals to gain in stature by taking sole responsibility! The good times were to pass, however, and in many ways the leaders of the profession had taken too much out and not put enough back. In those days, it was too easy to be respected, revered and indeed rewarded. The profession was tricked into not regulating itself in a way that society was soon to expect. I have myself always believed that apprenticeship in surgery was better than trial and error – a master and apprentice cannot reasonably or with justification be separated – and the NHS will no longer tolerate absentee landlords.

Working in 149 in the early days must have been fun, and real friendships existed between consultants who worked together and supported each other. Such friendships were cemented by the awe, ritual, tradition and hierarchy of the doctors' dining room. Like Gaul, it was historically divided into three

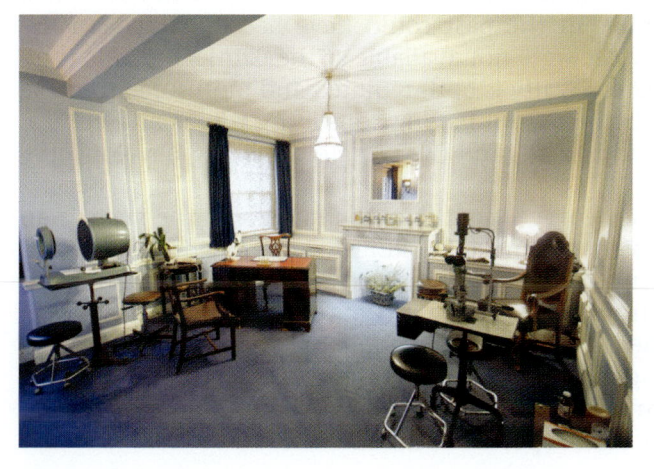

Figure 13.2 *A consulting room in 149 (see also frontispiece with author's office).*

parts: one for the consultants, one for administrative staff and another an overflow table. The lunch, or rather luncheon, was a three-course affair served by Aileen O'Donovan. One of the elder statesmen like Graham Hayward or Sir Francis Avery Jones took the head of the table with the doyen of Clinic general practitioners, Cuthbert Cain on the right (but not when a race meeting was within reach). Others like Roger de Vere and Walter Somerville were next, and below the salt came JP Williams, Garfield Davies and Hugo Rowbotham, who started his long association with the Clinic as resident medical officer. The juniors had to creep in and take their place appropriately. The food and camaraderie was a catalyst for an exchange of Clinic chat and undoubtedly served as a market place for referrals.

To some extent, close working relationships continue to exist as a result of the multidisciplinary approach to some forms of treatment – as in oncology – but on the whole consultants tend to arrive and depart with blinkers, focusing their activities on a narrow clinical goal of their own. This may change in the future, however, when consultants working in similar fields begin to form 'chambers' to allow time off and yet have cover from others – in addition to the benefits of concentrating complementary skills together.

To help keep the illusion of the past going, dinners for consultants were arranged two or three times a year in the late 80s and early 90s. These followed the 149 consultants' committees, which reported informally to the new chairman, James Ramsden, and his successor, Michael Abrahams. They were also useful for an exchange of ideas between the administration and clinicians. Sometimes one or two retired consultants were invited to these dinners to recount stories of their early days. Such fun and friendship, which helps build morale and team spirit, has now been put on one side by the new generation. Even the consultants' Christmas dinner is a thing of the past. How much they miss by regarding the Clinic merely as a resource centre of clinical excellence!

The rent that the consultants with rooms pay to the Clinic is in fact a 'service charge', and they are regarded as being in partnership with the Clinic. Failure to use the facilities in the past could have been justified on the grounds that certain services were not available at the Clinic, but this is no longer the case, and greater loyalty is both required and monitored to make the partnership work. The benefit of having consulting rooms and clinical facilities on one site is clear to all, and the principle is being developed by other private hospitals.

Included in the facilities enjoyed by the consultants over the years is an appointments office, which can make bookings when part-time users and their secretaries are absent or when full-time secretaries are away. Bookings are now becoming electronic and can be integrated with appointments in other departments of the Clinic if tests are required. Patients who enter 149 and the other consulting rooms provided by the Clinic are met by trained receptionists and shown to waiting rooms until they are summoned (often in person) by secretaries or the specialists themselves.

The front line – 149 Harley Street

As well as security personnel, there is an inevitable collection of closed-circuit television cameras, like nesting boxes around an arboretum. There was initial concern about this undermining patient confidentiality and privacy; however, the security aspect was seen to be paramount, and the tapes are viewed only by the security staff if a situation demands it. One of the more notorious recent events that needed security was the admission of President Pinochet of Chile after the war with Argentina over the Falkland Islands. He was admitted for a medical examination at the Clinic in October 1998 and underwent subsequent surgery. He was arrested in his room on the eighth floor and subsequently placed under guard while he recovered from the operation. The police wanted to set up a trial in his room, but the surgeon and chief executive rightly refused on the grounds that he was too unwell to appear before a magistrate.

Once the President was fit to be discharged, the chairman, chief executive and his surgeon had to confront the commissioner of the Metropolitan Police in the Clinic's boardroom to tell him that we were discharging the President, as was our right. They hastily agreed to move him elsewhere (to another hospital in North London), and he left via the tradesman's entrance by the rubbish bins. Later on, the chief executive of the hospital to which he was transferred called to ask how we managed to persuade the police to move him, as they wished to do the same. His arrest and the related detention cost the taxpayers £4m, of which the security costs at the Clinic were £1.2m. However, this paved the way for his release and return to Chile on grounds of ill health. A series of cartoons in the press recalls the national interest this situation provoked (Figure 13.3).

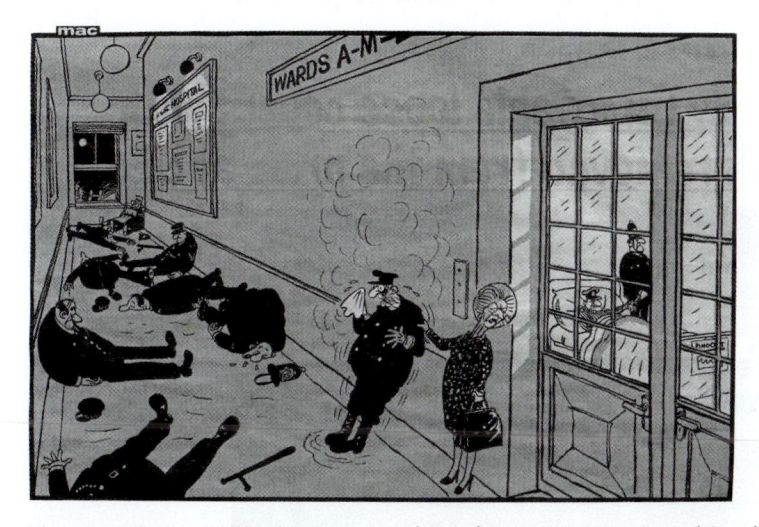

Figure 13.3 *'All right, Benson, this is his room. You carry him down to the car while I handbag the guard.' Reproduced with kind permission from Solo Syndication. Originally published in the Daily Mail, 23 October 1998.*

Our own royal family, enticed to the Clinic in more recent years by those such as Sir Richard Bayliss and Sir John Batten, used a discreet side door. This is managed with impeccable drill reminiscent of the Sovereign's Parade at Sandhurst. However, the Queen Mother always insisted, in her characteristic way, on having a friendly chat with all she came across – whether they had brooms or stethoscopes. Having opened the Clinic in 1932, I suspect she felt that she had a continuing special relationship. Visiting royalty from abroad is also managed with discretion and skill, as the secret admission of King Emmanuel of Italy showed.

The Terrace Restaurant (Figure 13.4) provides meals for patients' relatives if required, and Madame Tussauds is not far away for children in tow during the school holidays. The devotion of Arab families is reflected in the number of family members and mobile phones that accompany the patient. Their aromatic scent lingers until the next cleaning trolley patrols the corridor, but sometimes remains until the following morning.

Many receptionists and cleaning staff have come from abroad and find the Clinic a secure and friendly environment in which to work. They repay this by mastering English with enviable ease – often staying for many years and becoming appreciated by consultants and staff alike – as trusted servants in a gentlemen's club.

At the end of each day, most consultants leave their appointment books with the staff in the appointments office. Out of hours, urgent messages are passed on and less urgent ones left attached to the books for attention the next day. The staff are loyal in the extreme, even explaining that an absent specialist is away on a (golf) course (which is not, however, acceptable for gaining points for continuing professional development!).

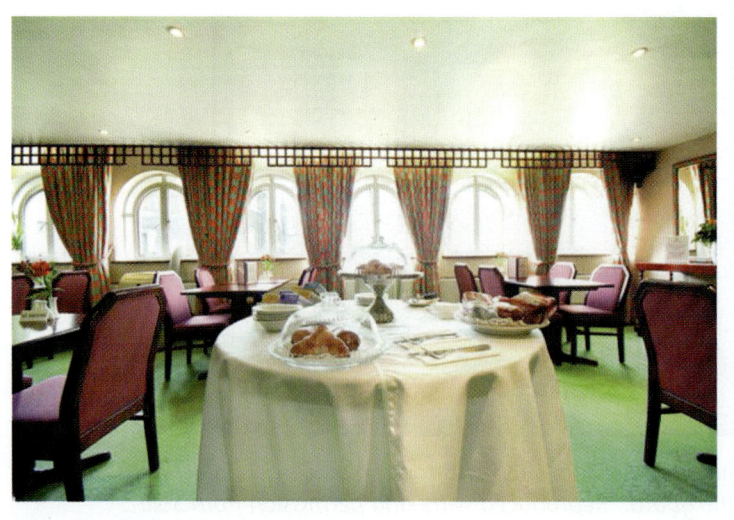

Figure 13.4 *Terrace restaurant.*

One of the longest surviving inhabitants of 149 is Dr D Geraint James, who started on St David's Day (1 March) 1959. This friendly, scholarly and ebullient Welsh physician was married to Dame Sheila Sherlock, a liver specialist of international acclaim, whose protégé Sir Anthony Dawson ultimately had rooms in the Clinic. Geraint James, who coined the phrase 'the intimacy of the Clinic', spent 40 years in 149, taking over the consulting rooms, secretary and furniture from Dr Forrest-Smith. Strangely, the clinical interests he had outside the Clinic – immunology, medical ophthalmology and postgraduate education – were never addressed by the Clinic, where, to this day, there is no medical library or even collection of publications by consultants. A commitment towards continuing professional development hopefully will develop. The department of nursing sets a fine example that clinicians should follow. The Clinic is now going to house and display the collection of the Hunterian Society, which is dedicated to the memory of John Hunter (1728–93), the founder of scientific surgery, and hopefully will be a catalyst for further medical collections. The rare books of the Hunterian Society, however, will continue to be housed in the Wellcome Institute, where there is a secure library.

As a prelude to future development at the Clinic, most consulting suites have been moved from 149 Harley Street and relocated to a dedicated outpatient development situated in 3–5 Devonshire Place, as well as 145 and 119 Harley Street (Figure 13.5). Within two years, further consulting rooms will be opened in 114–120 Harley Street. The 'rooms' are somewhat more

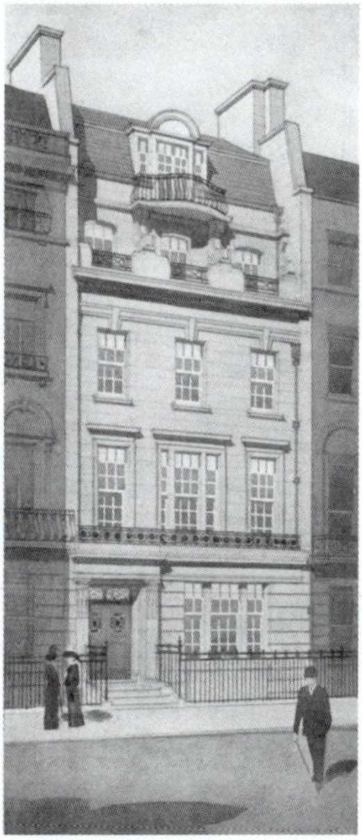

Figure 13.5 *119 Harley Street in 1911. Reproduced with kind permission from the City of Westminster Archives Centre.*

clinical and standardized, but they will still reflect some of the character and indeed clinical needs of the varying consultants. This, of course, is fitting for today's expectations. Communication between colleagues, laboratories and administration is increasingly electronic rather than personal. In order for this to be met, the ducts for computer trunking are more essential than a picture rail and room for diagnostic equipment more essential than a table for family photographs.

14
The heroes of old

Medicine depends greatly on apprenticeship for training and thus generates mentors and heroes. Intense loyalty and admiration are the by-products. Many of our national medical and surgical heroes were attached to the Clinic, which, despite the early financial problems, had appeared on the professional stage at the right time. Nowhere else in London (or even in England) could supply the needs of our 'heroes of old' as the apt and applicable phrase penned by Robert Browning (1812–99) would classify them! Distinguished physicians and surgeons fortunately were attracted to the Clinic.

It was a sellers' market, with patients almost queuing at the consulting room doors. This was the best that money could buy. The profession was, on the whole, honourable, despite their dependence on the trappings of town houses, staff and fine motorcars with chauffeurs. This can be matched now only by the odd plastic surgeon, anaesthetist, fertility doctor, dermatologist, gynaecologist or colorectal surgeon.

Many of those who have practised from the Clinic attracted and deserved justifiable fame and fortune. Some have left their names on equipment that they have developed – like Soutar's and McGill's tubes, Dunhill's forceps, Joll's retractor, Cheatle's forceps and Bonney's blue. Others, like Lord Dawson, Lord Horder, Lord Evans and Lord Webb-Johnson, have been prominent in our clinical and national life. Rowley Bristow and Manson Bahr, Dickson Wright, Laurance Abel, Ralph Marnham, Terrence Cawthorne, Francis Avery Jones, Ronald Bodley-Scott, Harold Gillies and Archie McIndoe are remembered for their expertise and pioneering clinical work. Demand was never short for those like Stanford Cade, Stephen Miller, Tudor Edwards, Naunton Morgan, Edward Muir, Rodney Maingot and Victor Negus, who were all leaders in their respective fields and many of whom were recognized with honours.

The traditions of these great men have more recently been continued by Norman Tanner, Ronald Furlong, Patrick Holmes Sellors, Tony Dawson and John Griffiths. The baton of apprenticeship has now passed to an equally distinguished group of specialists – more numerous in keeping with the need for an increased number of superspecialities and subspecialities.

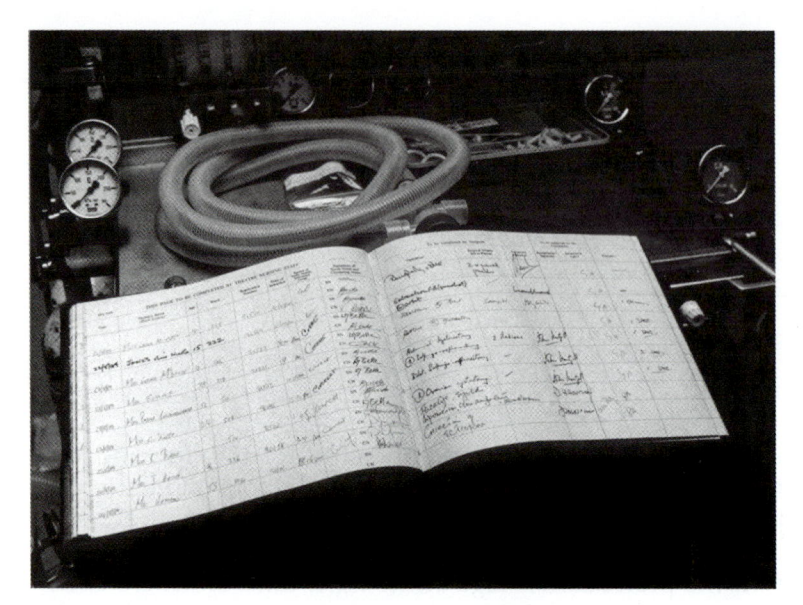

Figure 14.1 *Operating theatre record book.*

The great names I have listed will certainly be thought by some – or even many – to be incomplete. How can this criticism be overcome except by agreeing. I have given merely a dusting of chocolate on the surface of the large takeaway cup of cappuccino. I hope this will excite the devotees of medical history and biography to drink deeper. The Clinic has enabled all of these stars to come together under one roof in a royal command performance that started in 1932 and, like the Windmill Theatre, still continues day and night. Shakespeare wrote in *The Tragedy of Cymbeline, King of Britain*, Act IV 2, part of the song sung by Guiderius 'Fear no more the heat o' the sun':

> 'Thou thy worldly task hast done
> Home art gone and ta'en thy wages
> Golden lads and girls all must
> As chimney-sweepers, come to dust.'

By apprenticeship, however, and hand-in-hand with the developments taking place in the Clinic, the cancer centre and new consulting rooms, it will all continue without the final curtain coming down. Their activities are all recorded (Figure 14.1). How appropriate that a poet (Rudyard Kipling 1865–1936) alive at the time the Clinic was founded wrote:

> '"Let us now praise famous men...
> [The Holy Bible, Apocrypha, Ecclestiasticus 44.1]"
> ...And their work continueth.'

15
Spinning a yarn

There are always tales to tell in a community such as a hospital. Some are apocryphal; some notable through acknowledged but unchallenged exaggeration because of the enjoyment of the listener, who also is perhaps unwilling to deflate the ego of the narrator. The Clinic is no exception – dogs, motor cars and fishing tales sit comfortably between fact and fiction without challenge to their credibility.

As a young man, James Paterson Ross (later Sir James and President of the Royal College of Surgeons) used to assist Sir Thomas Dunhill at the Clinic. Having a young family and only an academic salary, he could not afford a motor car. At the end of one operating session, however, he was given £100 in cash by Sir Thomas – great riches at that time. As he walked down Regent Street from the operating theatre, he passed the Clinot showroom. The younger readers may not remember those classic French autos (which often looked rather like a junior char-à-bancs). He noticed one with a price ticket of £100, which just matched the money he had been given. He was tempted into the showroom. After a short while, he struck a deal for £95 (as the white-walled tyres were faded on one side). His elder son, Keith, who was Sir Thomas' godson, benefited also from his generosity. He was given a fine fishing rod rather than a motor car. Sir Thomas insisted on coming out onto the pavement of Harley Street in his dressing gown and slippers to give him a casting lesson. His younger brother Harvey (named after the American physician Harvey Cushing, who was a friend of Sir James) became a surgeon and had rooms in 149 Harley Street. In 1971, he sat with Sir Clifford Naunton Morgan and John Griffiths on the committee that was advising on improvements to the operating theatres.

One of Harvey Ross' illustrious patients at the Clinic had been Douglas Bader. On reflection, he regrets having parted with the cheque he received from Bader for the operation. It would have been a remarkable memento of the famous Battle of Britain pilot. He did, however, elect to remove the patient's sutures at home and noted that one of Bader's own trophies was a stiff white collar in his museum cabinet. It was inscribed 'From your great admirer Guy Gibson'.

Powerful and grand limousines have always attracted the attention of clinical specialists. I can remember a time when it was unusual to see many cars parked down the Street that were not Rolls Royces – many being chauffeur driven. This weakness for mechanical self-aggrandisement had early-on been ridiculed by Virginia Woolf, when she described Sir William Bradshaw's motorcar in her novel 'Mrs Dalloway.'

A surgeon who attracted attention with his amazing waistcoats and bright underpants in theatre in his early days practised what I shall describe as automobile deception. He used to hire a Rolls Royce and chauffeur to impress – and it clearly paid off. General practitioners found that the same practice was both self-enhancing and profitable. Indeed, the patients felt secure to have a show of automotive strength outside their houses when ill. A story is told of a general practitioner who still worked at the Clinic in the eighties and was late for a domiciliary visit when his car broke down. He incurred the displeasure of the patient. The next time he paid a visit he was tossed some keys and told that a new car (inevitably a Rolls Royce) awaited him in the basement. His astonishment at the generosity was later tempered by the fact that the value of the car was deducted from the legacy to him in the patient's will!

This year my bicycle will have been in continuous use by me for 60 years – only occasionally did I arrive on it at the Clinic. The chairmen, however, did give me a key to his garage, so that it could be hidden from view. I think he realized I was a potential public embarrassment, as I once was stuck after hours in the courtyard outside 149. This has very high railings, which are impossible to scale and the lock had jammed. I communicated my plight to passers-by in Harley Street, who told the porters at the Devonshire Place door. The porters thought it was a hoax. I, therefore, had to wait for the night watchman before being released. My anaesthetist used to arrive on a motorized scooter, and Dr Michael Zatouroff regularly arrived by bicycle from Highgate wearing an elegant polo hard-hat. How times have changed; seldom is a Rolls Royce or a chauffeur seen except for those bringing foreign dignitaries. An exception was King Hussein of Jordan, who was once spotted attending to a puncture on his own car, which had no chauffeur on that occasion.

Canine vignettes serve to demonstrate the holistic philosophy of the Clinic. I have always regarded dogs as an emotional deposit bank returning love and affection on demand – so unlike many friends and relatives. Dogs over the years have always had a definite but somewhat secretive and unrecognized relationship with the Clinic. I recently met an old lady who was delivered of her first child in the Clinic and had her Pekinese smuggled to her room in a hat box to give her comfort. I also knew an ear, nose and throat surgeon who, after-hours, used to come with his two Alsatians on his late night ward round. The house governor, Dick Kent, had a faithful Labrador called Tiger, which used to follow him up the back stairs to his flat.

My Labrador, Frisby, used to sit in my secretary's office at 149 and became a talisman for the patients – to the extent that some insisted that her photograph was in their room on admission. When Paul Getty was a long-stay patient, his dog was smuggled up the back staircase from time to time. A patient of mine once asked my secretary to arrange for the export of a dog from Harrods to the Middle East. The telegraphic address of Harrods in years gone by was 'Everything London'. The Clinic is similarly all-embracing.

The goings-on in the corridors of the Clinic did, famously, once come under close scrutiny from across Marylebone Road in Harley House. A disaffected relative decided to sue the Clinic. In order to obtain circumstantial evidence to add weight to her case, she rented a flat from which she had a good view of the Clinic and with binoculars and a notebook took up her post through the night and day. She hoped to record amorous exchanges between nurses and medical staff that distracted them from their duties. In 1959, Lady Hoare herself conducted part of the action for negligence (which was in connection with her husband, Sir Reginald Hoare's death). Ultimately, the story was regurgitated publicly in a trial to the delight of the press and the surprise of nurses and doctors in the Clinic. This was before the days of closed-circuit television, which now demands impeccable behaviour when in view of the cameras. Any indiscretions today require a little targeted reconnaissance beforehand – like those who know the whereabouts of the speed cameras on the roads into London. Both this case and one bought previously (1957) by Lady Wynn Parry (also for negligence, in which she claimed personal injury) were settled satisfactorily as far as the Clinic was concerned.

In the days before mobile phones and bleeps, we used to stay near the Clinic after an evening operating list to check that there were no postoperative complications before going home. We usually went to Campana – a much-favoured Italian restaurant in Marylebone High Street. It was popular not just for the asparagus, Barolo and carbonara but also because telephone sockets at the tables made it possible to have a telephone brought between courses to keep in touch with the Clinic.

Two distinguished rivals who focussed much of their private practices on the Clinic were Lord Dawson of Penn (Figure 15.1) and Lord Horder of Ashford (Figure 15.2). They attracted much notoriety in many fields – including the practice of euthanasia in their distinguished patients. The often-quoted satirical verse referring to the king's physician Lord Dawson's role in this respect (whether real or imaginary) is:

> 'Lord Dawson of Penn
> Has killed many men
> That is why we sing
> God Save the King!'

The present Lord Horder, however, affirms the original lines written by him in the 1930s as:[1]

> *'Lord Dawson of Penn*
> *Has killed many, many men*
> *But he doesn't do it to order*
> *Like Lord Horder'*

When he recited it at a family lunch one day, his father simply said, 'And you think that's funny?' Silence reigned for the rest of the meal.

Reference
1. Cook GC. The practice of euthanasia at the highest level of society: the Lords Dawson (1863–1945) and Horder (1871–1955). *J Medical Biography* 2006; **14**: 90–5.

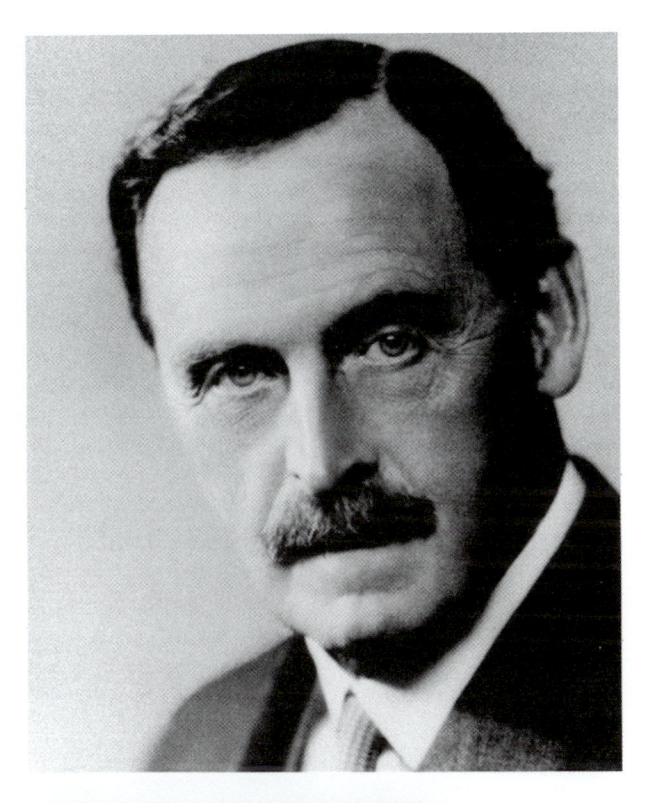

Figure 15.1 Lord Dawson of Penn. Reproduced with kind permission from the RSM Library.

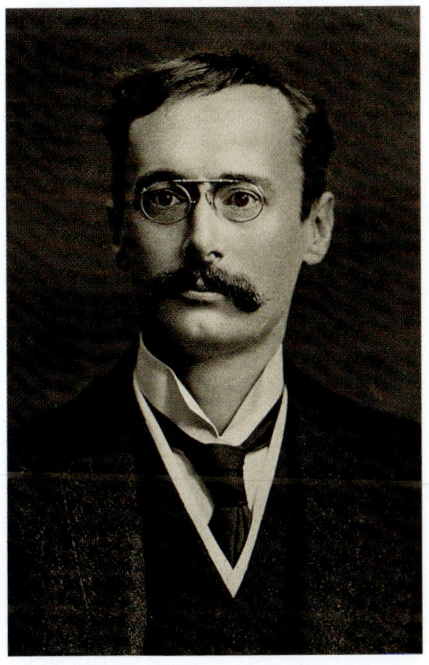

Figure 15.2 First Baron Horder of Ashford. Reproduced with permission from the Wellcome Trust Medical Photographic Library.

16
Theatres

A northern light is essential when artists immortalize their subjects (and themselves) on canvas, and so it was with the operating theatres at the Clinic. Initially situated on the eighth floor, landscape windows looked out over the plane trees on Marylebone Road and the slate roofs of Nash Terraces in Regents Park. The setting sun streamed down the corridor in the evening. It was a rarefied atmosphere of endeavour, dedication and occasional jealousy. The workplace was invaded by visiting surgeons, who brought their own instruments in monogrammed leather cases with drawers. They and their assistants were served by the Clinic's staff, who underpinned the itinerant surgical teams that visited from the outlying hospitals – some as far away as Leeds, whence the great Lord Moynihan came, leaving his patients in the care of trusted colleagues when he returned north at the end of the day. On arriving to change, the anaesthetist gave a fiver to the theatre orderly to fetch the patient for surgery. I expect the services of other members were recognized also – especially at Christmas.

With a variety of surgeons, it was necessary for the theatre sisters to be dominant and keep up discipline and standards. In those days, this was both expected and appreciated; we all knew where we stood and they ran a tight ship. Names such as Gillies (Figure 16.1), McIndoe (Figure 16.2), Dunhill and Moynihan (Figure 2.4) trod the boards in the theatres. There are those still living who had their anaesthetics administered by Sir Ivan McGill, who developed the intubation tube for anaesthetists. These tubes, a description of which was published in 1928, were used by him from the time the Clinic opened. He had his office in 149 Harley Street and worked closely with Sir Archibald McIndoe, who also consulted from there.

The rich and famous called the tune and eminent and innovative clinicians were easily enticed to minister to them. So it continued for many years. Patients sought the diagnostic experience and skills that the Clinic imprimatur guaranteed. The extent of the surgical procedures that needed to be undertaken was less easy to judge before the start of an operation than

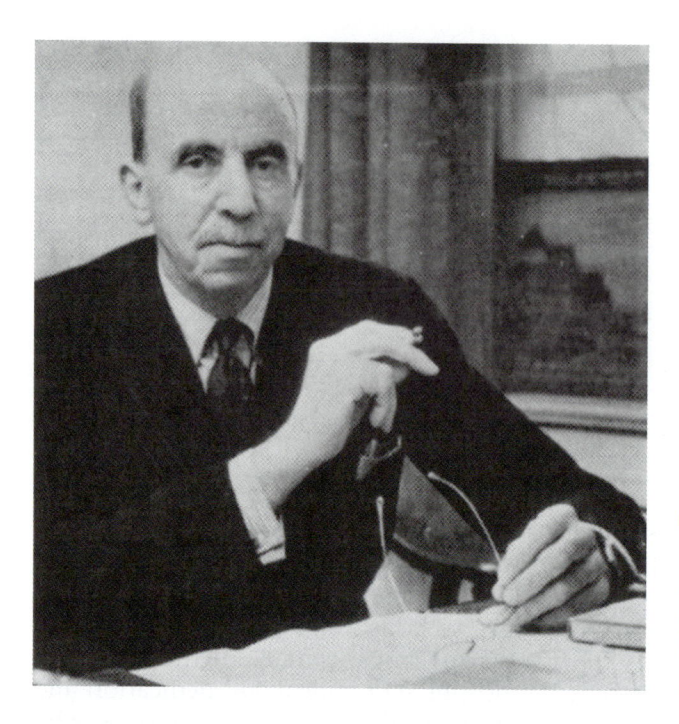

Figure 16.1
Sir Harold Gillies. Reproduced with kind permission from The London Clinic Medical Journal *1961;* **2***: 46.*

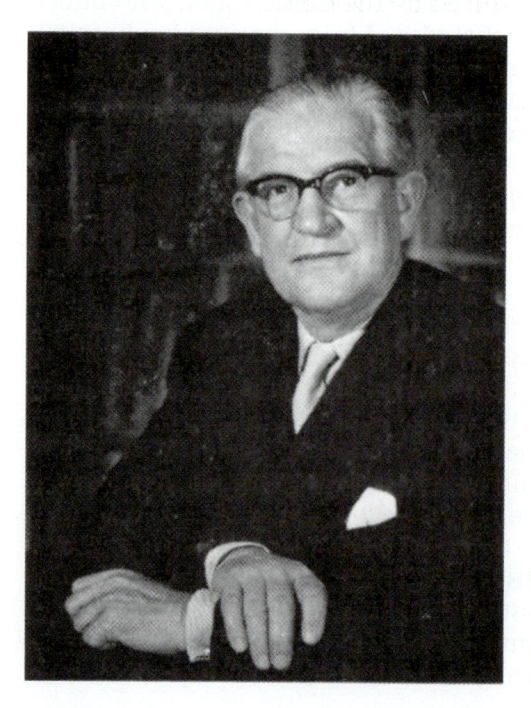

Figure 16.2 *Sir Archibald Hector McIndoe. Reproduced with kind permission from* The London Clinic Medical Journal *1960;* **1***: 25.*

today, when scans define the problem more precisely. An operation carried with it more of the spirit of pioneering exploration than is usually the case now. Risk, uncertainty and drama were not uncommon. A sense of theatre abounded, and this lingered on to form part of my early memories. When I was first at the Clinic, a senior colleague – the doyen of colorectal surgeons – was still operating at the age of 80 years. He took the precaution of admitting the patients under my name. He performed low colonic resections with the patient in the 'jack-knife position,' before turning them onto their back halfway through the procedure. This was a slightly unusual technique in my day, and he used to wander into the theatre in his colourful underpants and waistcoat in order to check that the patient was positioned correctly at the start of an operation. He employed large and long instruments with unusual skill and dexterity that would be rare to find nowadays.

On another occasion, a colleague had a complication and agreed to the family's request that he should be assisted by a surgeon they identified as the expert on that particular complication. This was on the basis of his having previously written a textbook on gastroenterology that was long out of date but still available in libraries in America. When the great man arrived, I was a little anxious. My worst fears were realized when he peered into the abdominal cavity and his spectacles fell into the wound. There was no time to wonder what would happen next – he simply returned them to their proper place and continued. All was well. In those days MRSA was not even a shadow on the horizon, as the prescribing of antibiotics had not been so abused and cleanliness was still next to godliness.

The theatres most famously served as a studio for Barbara Hepworth to study the anatomical shapes and forms that inspired the pictures she exhibited at the Lefèvre Galleries in 1946. She created, in mixed media, a series of drawings. The idea may have originated from Mr Norman Carpener, a surgeon in Exeter who himself was an amateur sculptor. The pictures verge towards the abstract and have a slightly misty and mysterious quality that captures the harmonious interactions of the doctors as they hover around the operating table (Figure 16.3). The detail of the drawing is concentrated in the hands and eyes of the surgeon. Rumour inevitably suggested that her relationship with the surgeon had acted as her inspiration.

In 1947, the Clinic decided to expand the operating theatres and they recruited staff (at five guineas a week). At that time, the facilities were very bare and basic (Figure 16.4). The anaesthetic rooms were devoid of equipment (which had to be brought by the visiting anaesthetist), although oxygen cylinders were provided. Anaesthetic gas cylinders were debited to the anaesthetist's accounts.

My anaesthetist used to bring his own cylinders with him in the seventies and eighties so as not to erode his profit margin too greatly and prejudice the upkeep on his enviable fleet of motor cars. Surgeons exercised similar economies when special techniques were being undertaken by supplementing their own instruments with ones borrowed from their NHS hospitals.

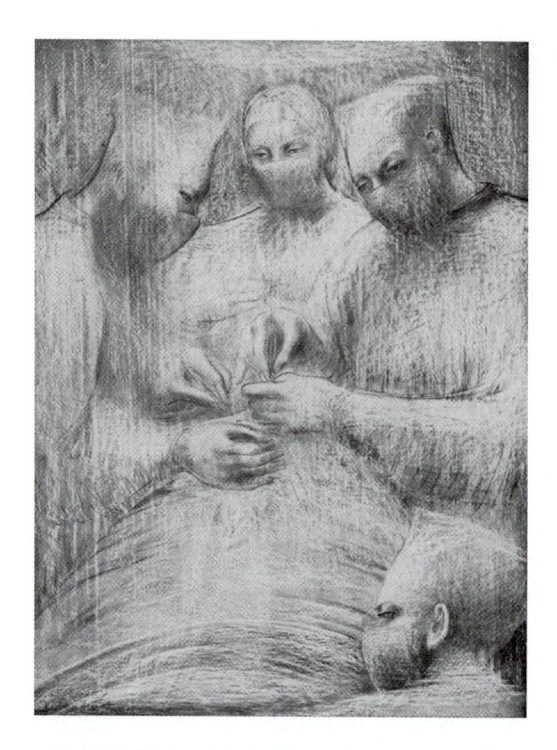

Figure 16.3 Concentration of Hands, no. 1, 1948, oil and pencil on plywood, 53.5 × 40 cm (British Council), Dame Barbara Hepworth. © Bowness, Hepworth Estate.

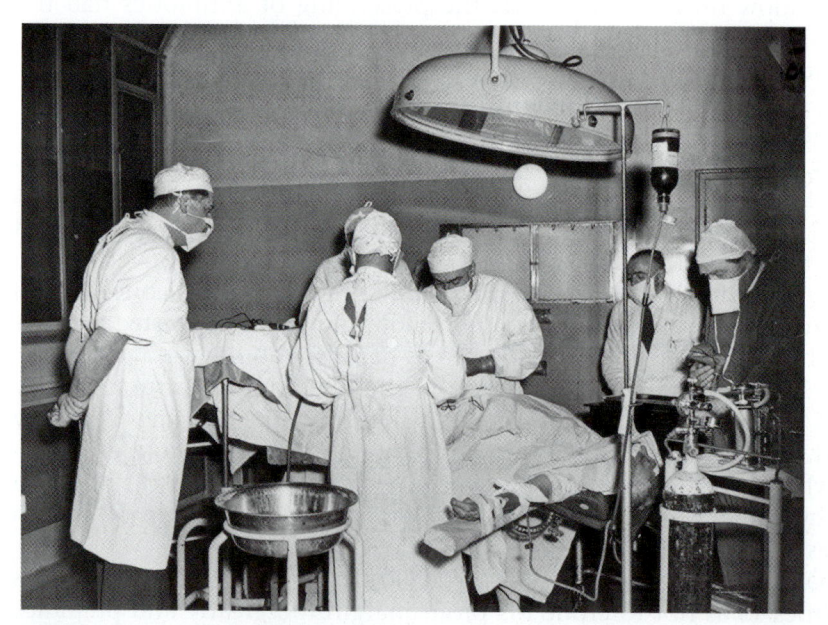

Figure 16.4 Operating Theatre before being relocated in the basement. Note the primitive anaesthetic equipment and surgeons not required to change completely from outdoor clothing.

Theatres **103**

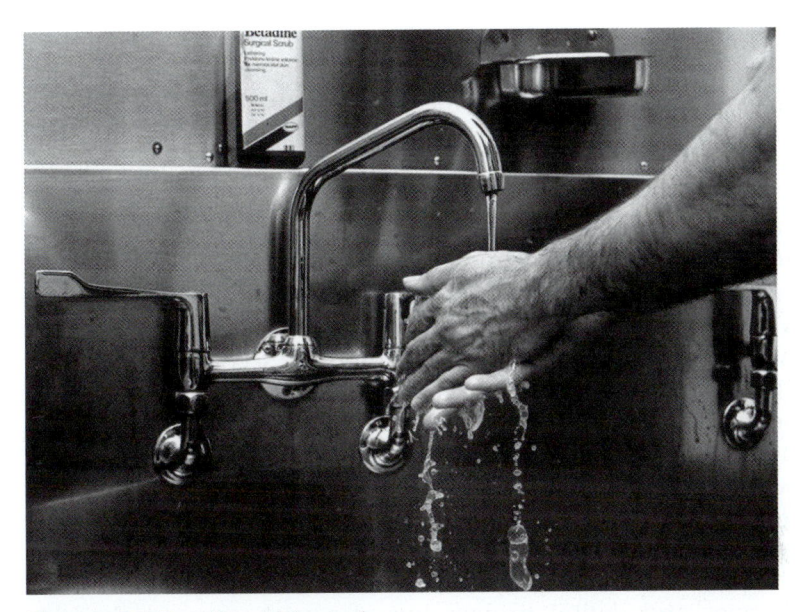

Figure 16.5 *'Scrubbing up'.*

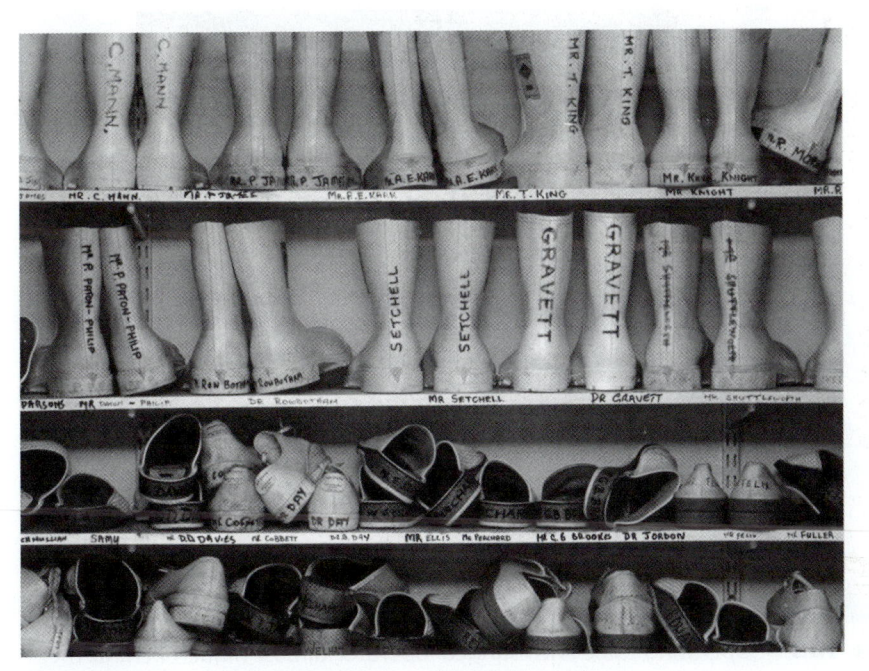

Figure 16.6 *Theatre boot room – 'ready for action'.*

Nowadays, surgeons expect and find all the necessary pieces of modern equipment and instruments ready when they arrive. They themselves, however, are beginning to be replaced in some situations by robotic techniques. The important innovation in this field is the installation of the da Vinci robotic surgical system – principally in the management of prostatic disease at present (Figures 16.7 and 16.8). This allows complex, fine, precise and technically reproducible skills to be offered to the patients, which leads to faster recovery and fewer complications. These techniques undoubtedly will spread to other fields.

Instruments for conventional operations are pre-packaged for each operation and appear with deceptive ease. Behind the scenes in the central supply department, cleaning, counting, packaging and sterilization take place. The possibility of linking this department with the needs of other hospitals and moving it offsite is being investigated. There is not yet computerized control, as on the shelves at a supermarket, but I expect that will come. Until then, instruments are counted in, rechecked and counted out with the swabs. Nowadays, the ritual of a patient entering and leaving the theatre is accompanied not only by a check list, an identity bracelet and details of allergies and dental bridges but also with a comprehensive preoperative informed consent and an indelible mark to confirm the side of certain procedures. An anaesthetic record printout, which includes vital

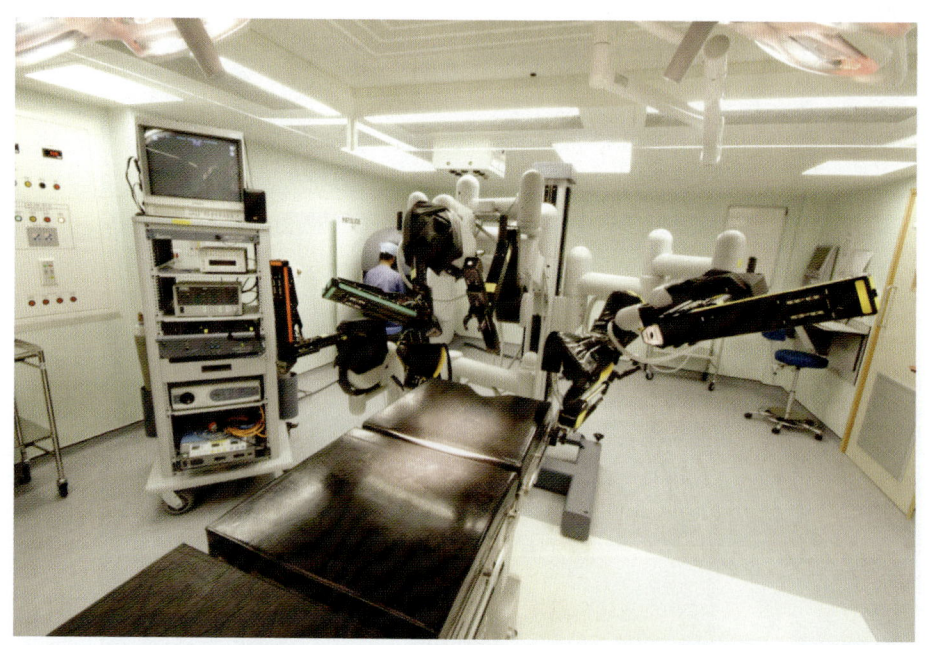

Figure 16.7 *Operating table with surgical operator almost hidden behind the robotic arms.*

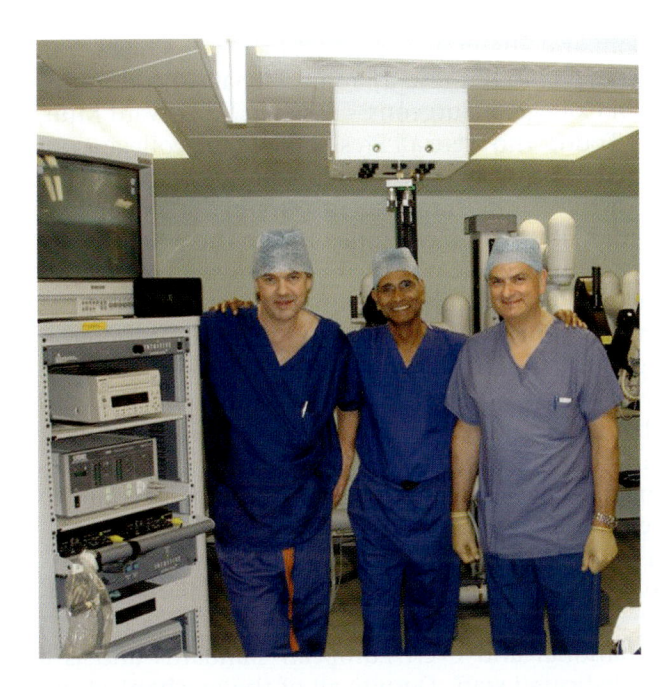

Figure 16.8 *Part of the da Vinci robotic team posing with their new toy! Professor Roger Kirby, Mr Krishna Patil and Dr Peter Amoroso.*

signs, accompanies each patient back to the ward, and a video record is becoming a legal requirement for some operations to protect the patient, surgeon and Clinic.

Today the theatres are in the basement. They had, in fact, previously been there for a short period in the Second World War as a security measure but afterwards had returned to the eighth floor. Relocation to the basement involved several years of planning. In 1971, a subcommittee under the chairmanship of Sir Clifford Naunton Morgan was set up with a younger colleague, Harvey Ross, and an anaesthetist, AJH Hewer. The terms of reference also embraced investigating the provision of intensive care, sterilizing facilities, recovery and minor surgery. Even then the problem of staffing was considered, as well as the ever-increasing cost of equipment and the need for air-conditioning. One of the major hurdles in the planning was to satisfy the Greater London Council's Fire Department that the means of escape from the basement and smoke control were adequate.

Everything has become more complicated and controlled in the theatres – not only in the field of equipment innovation but also with new techniques and health, safety and risk issues including both laser safety and patient confidentiality. This would not allow any intrusions such as those artistic ones by Barbara Hepworth to take place today! Nine essential checks are in place, including identity, clearance from the criminal records bureau and, more recently, documentation showing hepatitis B status before assistants can even enter the operating theatre complex.

The surgeons' coffee room and changing rooms over the years have doubled not only as a professional club but also as an unofficial subcommittee of the Council of the Royal College of Surgeons – as when Sir Edward Muir, Sir Alan Parkes and Sir Ian Todd, who were all Presidents of the college, continued to focus their practice on the Clinic. They would surely now be proud that the theatres in the Clinic have recently trained 12 operating department practitioner graduates who have gone off into the world.

The theatre office can accommodate three clerks and a sister. As they sit behind plate glass looking into the busy theatre corridor, it is never clear to me whether they or we are looking into or out of an aquarium. Whichever it is, they are clearly the goldfish and we the restless sharks looking for prey. Their accommodation is certainly a change from the small broom cupboard that served as an office before. The way the staff twist and turn to support the clinical need by fitting in emergencies and over-running lists requires vision, tolerance and ingenuity – ingredients we have perhaps come to expect without enough gratitude over the years.

A storekeeper and assistant are now inevitably supported by a computer. The stock held, including orthopaedic prostheses, is greater than in the central stores. The hospital sterilization and decontamination unit (HSDU) meets all national, international and even European standards and is a centre of excellence with dedicated staff. Despite all of the mechanization, the autoclaves are still named Dilys and Beverley after the wives of the engineers who installed them.

Intensive therapy, high dependency and progressive care units

In 1983, Michael Jenner as house governor realized the need to plan an intensive therapy unit (ITU) and approached Jack Tinker, director of the ITU at the neighbouring Middlesex Hospital. A planning group was set up, and a three-bed unit initially opened on 1 January 1989 in the basement close to the theatre complex. This was a general ITU fully equipped in terms of monitoring and support equipment. The patients retained their rooms on the nursing floor. In addition to dedicated nursing staff, an additional post of resident medical officer was created. The unit opened under the direction of Jack Tinker. From 1999, dedicated anaesthetists (Dr Aubrey Bristow and Dr John Goldstone) were in charge. A need was developing for patients to progress from the unit to somewhere within the Clinic before returning to their own rooms, so a high dependency unit (HDU) was opened on the third floor, with more acutely ill patients being cared for in the progressive care unit (PCU) (Figure 16.9). Patients progress from the ITU to the PCU, which was developed on the third floor. Monitoring includes not only the latest cardiac and respiratory monitoring but also close liaison with the laboratory for chemistry and other physiological

Theatres

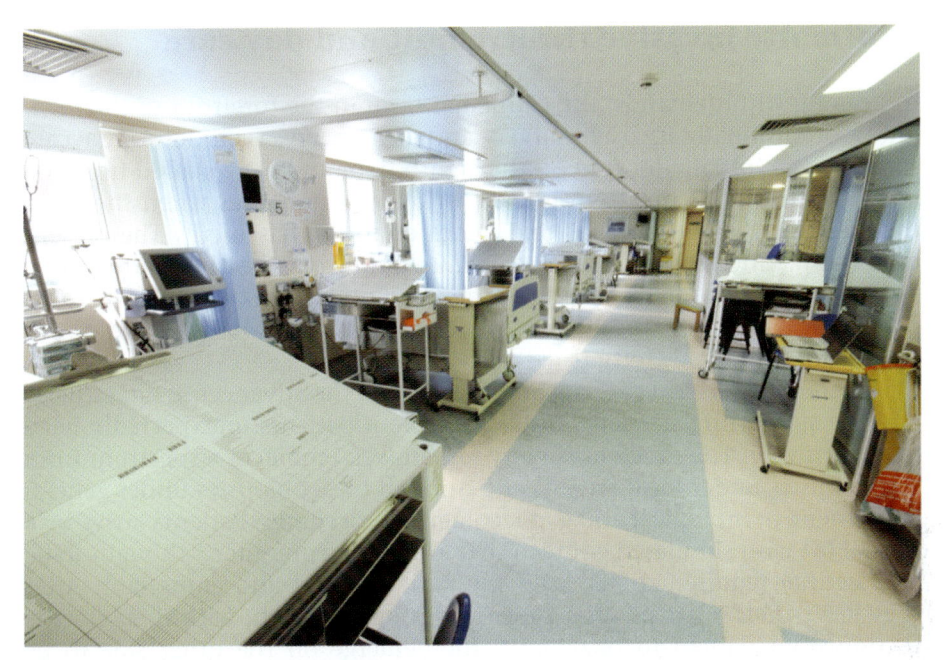

Figure 16.9 *Progressive care unit.*

measurements. By creating these units, the need for individual specialist nursing in rooms, which had, in the past, been the routine for major surgery, was largely superseded. The specialist nursing in rooms had been expensive – both in personnel and equipment – and quite rightly fell outside many of the non-comprehensive insurance policies that patients had taken out. The new system led to a more efficient use of personnel and the development of a special expertise that greatly helped postoperative management. An almost seamless transition could be achieved from the theatre to the patient's own room. The range of cases is wide, including gastrointestinal and prostate, spinal fusion, craniotomy, renal transplant and immunosuppressed patients. Some – mainly from the Middle East – are admitted directly to the unit.

An effective unit requires both a team spirit and a steady flow of patients needing such services. A critical mass must therefore feed into the system in order to maintain standards. For this reason, smaller hospitals find it difficult to develop units that can function with the sort of precision required, which is reminiscent of a pit stop in a Formula One race. The Clinic, unlike some other private institutions, is large enough to support such a unit. With nursing staff in training, and a 24-hour rotation of consultants, cover by doctors and nursing staff trained in intensive therapy can be provided. This level of care is continued after patients return to their own rooms ('ITU without walls') and after patients' discharge with outreach nursing care.

Minimally invasive theatre unit and day care

In keeping with demands, the Clinic has been in the forefront of the revolution of minimally invasive surgery and day surgery. Facilities for daycare surgery were initially located on the eighth floor and were staffed from the main theatres. This theatre was used for quite major cases when the main theatres were being upgraded and relocated to the basement. The present unit was planned so that specialist teams could work together and develop a service that could meet the special requirements of this newly developing discipline. The current unit was opened in May 1995 by the wife of our benefactor John Paul Getty II.

This trend in clinical care depends heavily on the advances in anaesthesia and the supporting specialist units available if patients unexpectedly need overnight care. The range of surgery undertaken embraces a spectrum from skin biopsies under local anaesthetic through breast biopsies under general anaesthetic to urological and gynaecological procedures. Patients arrive by a special lift with simulated goldfish that are fed by computer – thought to be an essential requirement to keep the patients calm and compliant. After they leave their relatives, they proceed through the unit, with their clothes accompanying them in bags, until they emerge on the other side to be reunited with relatives who are now sitting comfortably sipping coffee and reading magazines. The unit is suspended within the Clinic on the third and fourth floors, sitting like an embryo within its mother, the Clinic – self-sufficient and self-contained but dependent. It is indeed an embryo that is destined to grow and continue to absorb much work that formally depended on inpatient admissions.

17

Radiology, radiotherapy and imaging

Radiology and radiotherapy

An entry from 1946 in the minutes of what was then called the board of governors suggests that counsel's opinion as to whether the Clinic was entitled to provide x-ray services to outpatients must be sought – presumably in view of the original Howard de Walden lease, which gave permission for 'a Clinic and nursing home'. Outpatient services were perhaps not anticipated originally but happily were allowed to develop in an area where retail services up and down the elegant residential street inevitably would be frowned on. The x-ray department ultimately was opened in January 1948. By then, three radiologists – Drs J Bull, E Allen and WO Macfeat – received £50 a year and £250 of expenses. The departmental budget approved in 1949 was for £12,530.2.8p. The financial relationship of the radiologists with the Clinic was always under review and, indeed, a continuing subject of concern, but a share of the profits that amounted to £3,350 was distributed between them in 1950. Aynsley Bridgland reviewed the whole of the department in 1951 and intervened, as there was not only difficulty in patients securing appointments but dissension among the radiologists, problems with the purchase of materials and the engagement of staff without authority. The initial explanations by Drs Allan and Macfeat to the board did not resolve the matter immediately.

Tacked on to the continuing problems of the radiology department was the possible development of a radiotherapy department. This first mention appeared in the minutes as a proposal in 1952. In July of that year Dr WM Levitt negotiated a 70% share of the profits of such a department, but that might have been a little premature, as by October the committee was still waiting for proposals for staff appointments. The matter had to be deferred further. Negotiations about the radiotherapy and cobalt department continued and ultimately (in 1957) it was proposed that Dr Levitt be regarded as an employee of the Clinic and Dr RJ Dickinson as director of radiotherapy.

Despite the difficulties in integrating the new service with the more traditional aspects of treatment within the Clinic, patients were being treated. There are records of an irradiation protection committee to test the efficacy of protection arrangements and also of the purchase of 339.5 curies of cobalt-60 from the United Kingdom Atomic Energy Authority. Repairs to the cobalt unit in 1967 cost £7,500 and the wisdom of continuing to offer this treatment was questioned. In 1970, £400 was recorded as being spent on maintenance of the cobalt machine. The feasibility of continuing to offer radiotherapy was ultimately not practicable, however, with the need for higher doses, linear accelerators and consequently greater radiation protection. In 1971, patients were transferred to St Bartholomew's Hospital, the Royal Free Hospital or St Mary's Hospital. The phoenix of radiotherapy is destined to rise from the ashes of the original initiative, however, in the new comprehensive cancer clinic being developed in Devonshire Place.

Radiology continued to flourish and develop into the present day department, which embraces all the modern techniques of radiology, ultrasound and invasive procedures. This has evolved over the years from the small beginnings in 1948. The visiting staff who have provided a service over the years have husbanded the developments that have enabled us to reach today's level of sophistication.

In 1970, the head of the department was Dr W Ogilvie Macfeat, who was, of course, in post at the inception of the department. He lived in the Clinic in a luxurious flat that overlooked Harley Street and was fastidious in his work as well as the selection of staff. The distinguished neuroradiologist Dr James Bull, was also on the staff when the department was started. He had been a prisoner of war, escaping the slaughter of patients, nurses and medical staff by the Japanese at the Alexandra Hospital in Singapore by hiding in a cupboard. A happy coincidence was that Dr Robert Dick shared duties at the Clinic with Dr Bull. Dick's father, a surgeon, and Dr Bull had both been prisoners of war in Changi, Singapore. This bond was rekindled 40 years later when Dick the younger undertook routine investigations after Dr Bull had finished the esoteric angiograms and myelograms. Thereafter the senior man repaired to Brown's Hotel, where he used to stay elegantly overnight before returning to Henley the next day.

Although Dr Macfeat ran a very traditional department – even down to the furniture in the changing rooms – he was not averse to informal clothing (pale blue short-sleeved Aertex shirts for staff). However, new techniques, such as percutaneous cholangiograms, he delegated to the younger members such as Dr Dick. His own standards were legendary. One always had to wait until the final follow-through picture before passing a comment or communicating the result to Sir Francis Avery Jones, with whom he worked closely. Along with his colleagues Drs Hatley and Howlett and the remarkable superintendent radiographer Helen Warner, he headed an impressive team. The discipline and regimentation of the department probably owed something to the early influence of the hairbrush used on his feet

Radiology, radiotherapy and imaging **111**

by his mother and kept by him as a symbol of his upbringing – although he had long since lost his hair.

One radiological investigation slow to be provided by the Clinic was mammography. This was simply through lack of space and has now been addressed. It does show, however, the issues that have to be considered by those involved in strategic planning and how difficult it is to overcome the constraints of space and finances. What is required and how any need can best be met has to decided – while keeping an eye on the bottom line of the accounts. This is something that politicians also find notoriously difficult in the provision of NHS facilities with limited resources.

Today, the department has 45 clinical staff and 62 consultants, including electromyographists, vascular specialists and gynaecological radiologists. In 2006, there were 33,129 radiology procedures. The Clinic has a total of 17 procedure rooms, including those in 5 Devonshire Place (Figure 17.1).

Delivery of healthcare demands continuing evolution and change. The new techniques of ultrasound complement the traditional x-rays, and invasive investigative radiology walks hand in hand here and in the new facility in 5 Devonshire Place, which allows techniques such as needle biopsies and embolization when required.

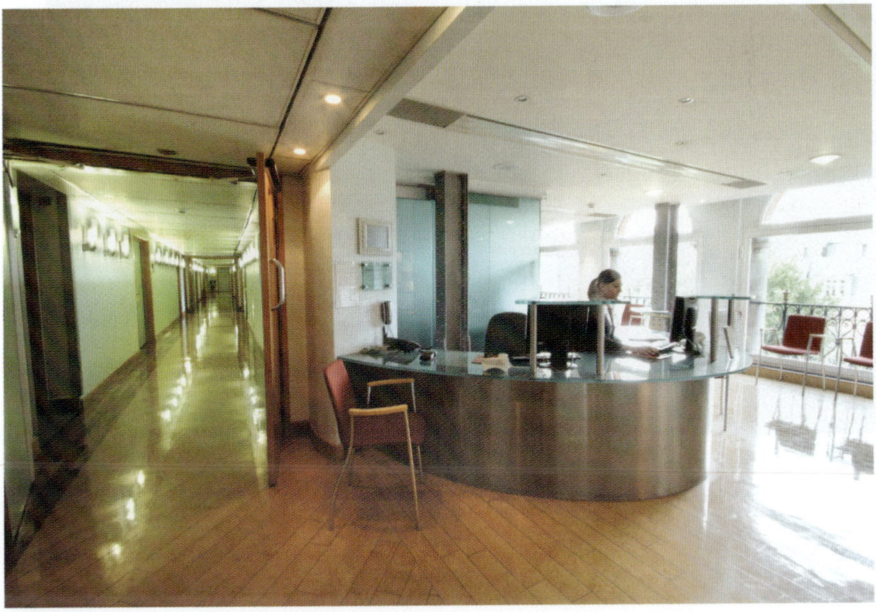

Figure 17.1 *X-ray Reception Desk.*

Imaging

On the same floor is the imaging department, facilities for computed tomography (CT) and magnetic resonance imaging (MRI) (Figure 17.2). The roots of this department date back to 1989, when Dr (now Professor Dame) Janet Husband and Tiba Seear were collaborating at the BUPA Medical Centre in the Pentonville Road. The disadvantage of this site for a private medical investigation centre was apparent in the difficulty of marketing a considerable capital investment in a rather depressed area of London. The Clinic was approached by this enterprising pair, who saw the opportunity of capturing a wide referral base. A deal was struck with the ladies; in return for space the equipment was provided and installed by them. The first patient scanned was in 1989. MRI was added in 1991 to what was already a flourishing department which was officially opened by Princess Margaret in October of that year. Such a rising star in the diagnostic galaxy could not be left out in the cold, and the imaging department was acquired by the Clinic in 1999 – a marriage of convenience but also made in heaven.

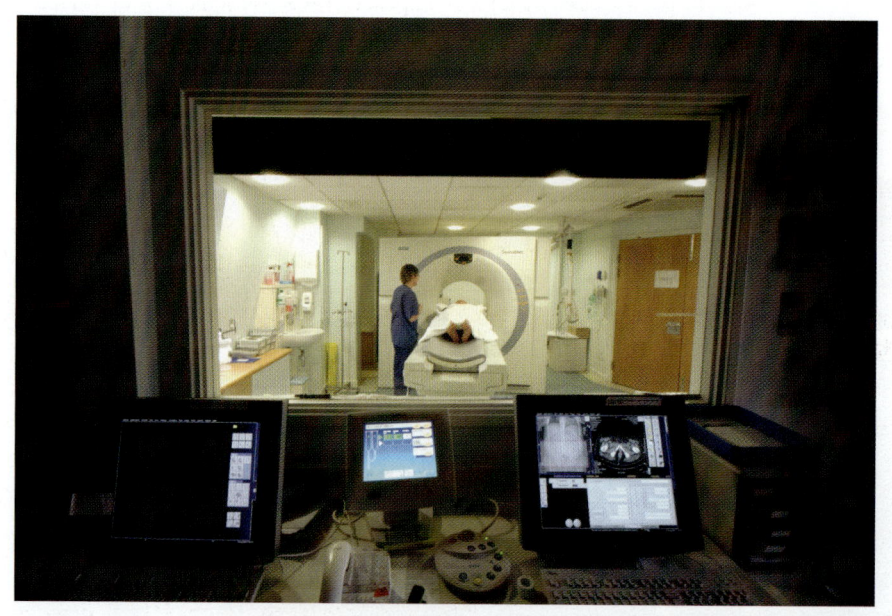

Figure 17.2 *Control room and computed tomography scanner.*

18
Endoscopy

The concept of truly flexible gastroscopy originated from Imperial College, London, in 1954, with Hopkins and Kapany's paper in the *Lancet* describing the feasibility of image transmission down a bundle of glass fibres and coining the term 'fibrescope'. Rigid oesophagoscopes, bronchoscopes and 'semi-flexible' gastroscopes had for many years been in occasional use in the operating theatres, but they were cumbersome and had obvious limitations, including the inability to bend around the stomach into the duodenum to diagnose ulcers. Clinically useful flexible endoscopes eventually arrived, from American and Japanese manufacturers, in the late 1960s. In common with other private hospitals, the earliest days of flexible endoscopy depended on individual enthusiasts bringing their own fibreoptic gastroscopes, colonoscopes or bronchoscopes to examine individual patients booked into the operating theatres at the top of the hospital or the x-ray department.

By the early 1970s, flexible endoscopy was supplementing or supplanting plain radiography as a routine diagnostic procedure thanks to the advantages of colour pictures and biopsy, cytology or aspiration specimens. The first private sector endoscopy unit in the country was opened in 1975 in Harley House opposite the Clinic by Mr John Chalstrey (a Bart's surgeon, who was later knighted as the first medical Lord Mayor of London) with his friend Dr Tony Fenton Hill (a GP with experience of endoscopy and family commercial resources). Their 'panendoscopy' facility in the basement of Harley House was excellent and demonstrated the advantages of a well-equipped daycare endoscopy service run by specialist nurses for visiting consultants and their patients.

With the Clinic's operating theatres transposed to the basement in 1977, some space seemed to be free. Christopher Williams recalls that he and Peter Cotton persuaded the house governor, Mr Michael Jenner, to allocate an area for endoscopy adjacent to the new X-ray department at the top of the hospital. This became the first hospital-based endoscopy unit in the private sector in the UK. Dr W Ogilvie MacFeat, director of radiology and a gastrointestinal specialist enthusiastic about having younger people in his department, was supportive of the idea. The result was a thriving single-room endoscopy unit staffed by two endoscopy nurses (initially Helen Michelsen, then Aileen Maloney and Wanda Gorecki) and a secretary. There were three small trolley cubicles in which patients could change and recover afterwards. This tiny facility and tight-knit team gave an efficient service despite the need for consultants to change and dictate their reports while hidden away in a miniscule storage cupboard in the corner of the endoscopy room. Instrument cleaning and disinfection was careful but basic. The lead endoscopists initially supplied their own instruments, which they also used for 'peripatetic endoscopy' when called to other hospitals. The decision that the Clinic should own all instrumentation was made early on in the best long-term interests of all concerned. This move ensured that only skilled endoscopists were accepted to use the facility, because of the need to protect the small stock of instruments – initially fragile as well as

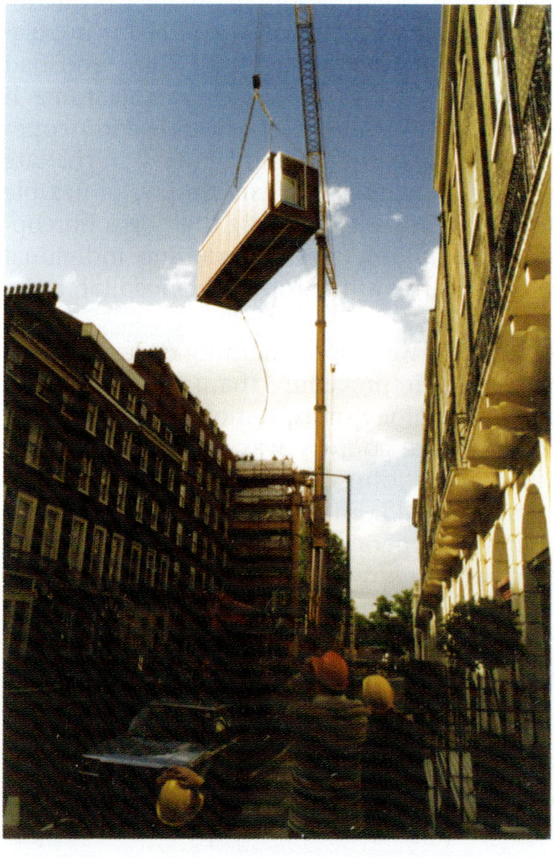

Figure 18.1 *The temporary unit being lifted into position over the roof to be suspended on the west side of 149 from the seventh floor.*

Endoscopy 115

expensive – and in the best interests of patients and referring practitioners. The combination of high standards, morale and friendliness in this small team established a reputation.

In September 1996, after prolonged lobbying (and two years in a temporary building precariously mounted seven floors from the ground (Figures 18.1 and 18.2)), a three-room unit with 11 patient cubicles and reception, waiting, sterilizing, nursing and storage areas was built over a substantial area of flat Clinic roof.

The new endoscopy unit was, most fittingly, ceremonially opened by the Lord Mayor of London, Sir John Chalstrey. The unit was styled elegantly throughout thanks to major input from the suppliers of the endoscopes (KeyMed for Olympus Optical, Tokyo), with the technical areas showplaces for ergonomic design and having the most advanced endoscopic equipment (Figure 18.3). The service expanded progressively to more than 9,000 patients annually (including occasional bronchoscopies), with 20 sessional consultants (many regarded as leaders in their specialty in the UK), five receptionists, 18 nursing staff (with Wanda Gorecki in charge) and two instrument technologists. Demand for gastrointestinal endoscopy continues to increase, currently fuelled by requirements for colon screening. Yet another 'new endoscopy unit' is planned therefore – an evolutionary cycle with which those involved with the Clinic are familiar.

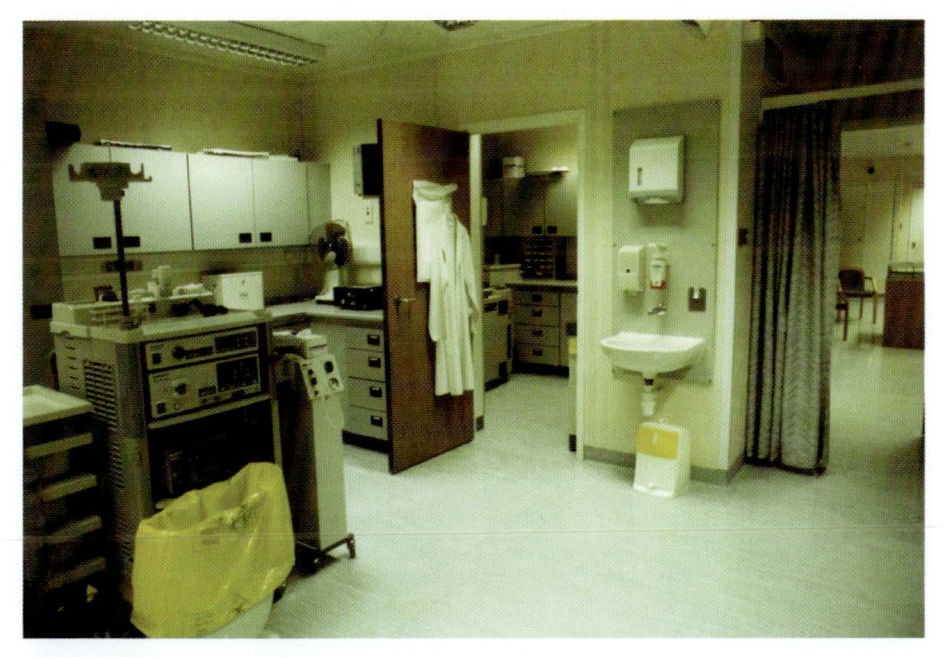

Figure 18.2 *Temporary endoscopy unit.*

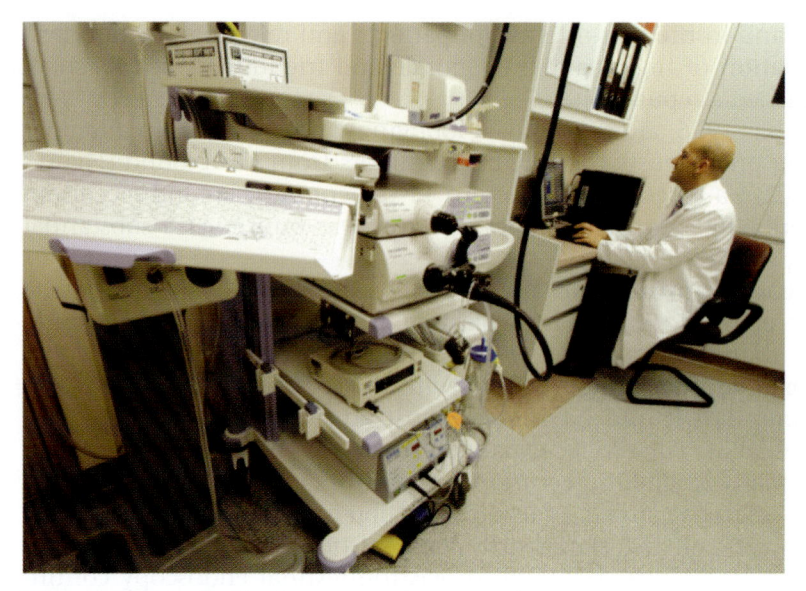

Figure 18.3 *Inside the new endoscopy unit.*

19

Pathology and pharmacy

Pathology

As diagnostic skills increased hand-in-hand with the new era of measurement in medicine, so the pathology department had to grow. The possibility of incorporating the new department in part of the development taking place in 18 Devonshire Place was raised. This was proposed as early as 1948, some ten years before Dr Spence, director of pathology, was looking for new staff in 1958 to expand the department. Before the days of automated equipment, even more than today, the quality of the work depended on the excellence of technical staff. They were largely recruited from NHS hospitals, lured by better working conditions and the knowledge that they could provide a good service without cutting corners and receive a slightly enhanced take-home pay. Bob Crawford was the chief technician in histology at this time, with Don Macmillan in bacteriology, Duncan Woods in haematology (under Dr Kirkpatrick) and Mike Jennings, who replaced Gordon Hartman when he went to Chelsea College to study for a technical diploma. A strong tradition of continuing education among the staff underpinned the enthusiasm and quality of their work. Mike Jennings did a diploma at Chelsea College in microbiology and eventually obtained a PhD at London University – a very creditable performance that was encouraged by the Clinic. The team of technicians were led by Dr Tony Chaazn in haematology and Dr Roman Jakobski in bacteriology and histology, who kept up the standards of the Clinic with a rolled umbrella and a bowler hat. Jacobski was Polish and had trained in medicine in Beirut during the Second World War, which was where the Polish Medical School had been evacuated during those difficult years. He was able to provide an excellent service across a wide range of pathological disciplines. The newly established College of Pathologists, however, brought with it the realization that more specialization was essential as knowledge of disease progressed. Not only was this required between the four sections of pathology but also within the sections themselves.

Dr Basil Morson, consultant pathologist at the Colorectal Hospital, St Mark's, City Road, was brought into the Clinic by his colorectal surgical colleague Mr John Griffiths, who needed specialist pathological opinions in this field. Thereafter, many other specialists, including Dr Peter Trott, the internationally renowned breast cytopathologist, were appointed, which reflected the increasingly complicated nature of diagnostic pathology.

Dr Kirkpatrick had made a very positive contribution to biochemistry by devising a method of measuring protein-bound iodine that preceded the new range of radioimmunoassay tests that were being ushered in. One of the technicians, John Howard, built a spectograph for measuring trace metals, which was even used to measure levels of chromium in wine. It was decided to computerize the laboratory around this time, and £10,000 was invested in the project. With Mike Worthington and later Ron Waite, the information technology revolution started in the Clinic. When Dr Roman Jakobski retired in 1985, the laboratory retained the leather-bound ledgers in which he had meticulously recorded reports stretching back to 1974. From then on, the laboratory entered the electronic era.

The laboratory now handles up to 14,000 specimens per year and has clinical pathology accreditation (CPA) (Figure 19.1). Three colorectal pathologists have replaced Dr Basil Morson, who retired in 1992, and there are now lymphoma, gynaecological and endocrine experts, and specialist opinions in dermatology. These were provided initially by Professor Wilson Jones until his retirement in 2000. The need for a wide range of experts in neuropathology, head and neck pathology and osteopathology demands that visiting expertise is required during the working week. Online communication greatly assists the delivery and checking of pathological reports when the experts return to their NHS hospitals during office hours.

Microbiology has developed since the appointment of Professor Brian Lacey in 1978 and is now a major field. An expertise in hospital infection is essential with the prevalence and publicity given to such problems as the bacillus responsible for Legionnaire's disease (*Legionella pneumophila*) and MRSA. No account of microbiology at the Clinic would be complete without mention of Geoff Phillips, who was principal microbiologist and laboratory manager for more than 20 years. His persistent attention to detail had given the microbiology department renown within the independent sector, and this tradition lives on today (Figure 19.2).

The routine haematological services that were in the hands of Dr Tony Chaazan and Dr Alan Salsbury in the 1980s, including blood transfusions, have now developed into a major specialty that covers a wide range of haematological diseases including leukaemia. In July 1984, the first bone marrow transplant was undertaken on a general ward. In January 1985, Dr Peter Gravett, previously consultant haematologist to the Royal Army

Pathology and pharmacy **119**

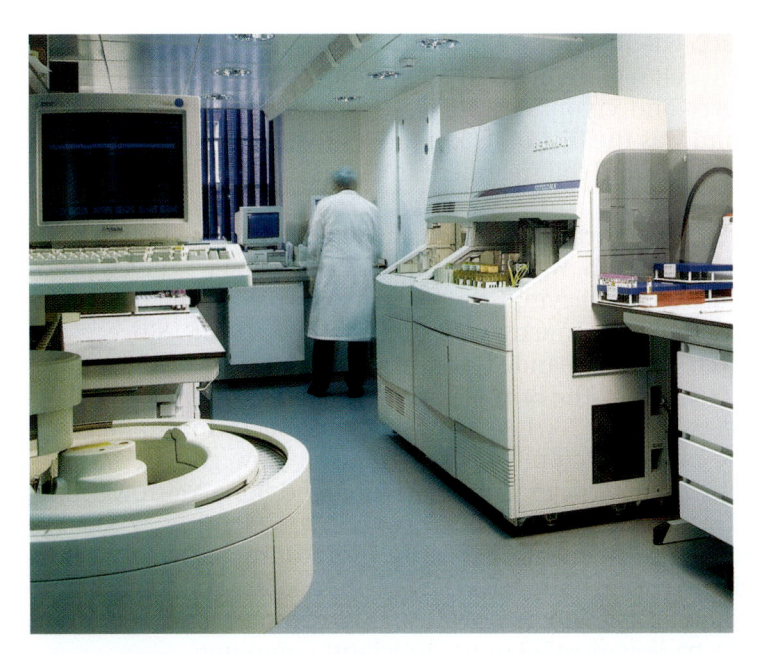

Figure 19.1 *Pathology Department – computerized equipment.*

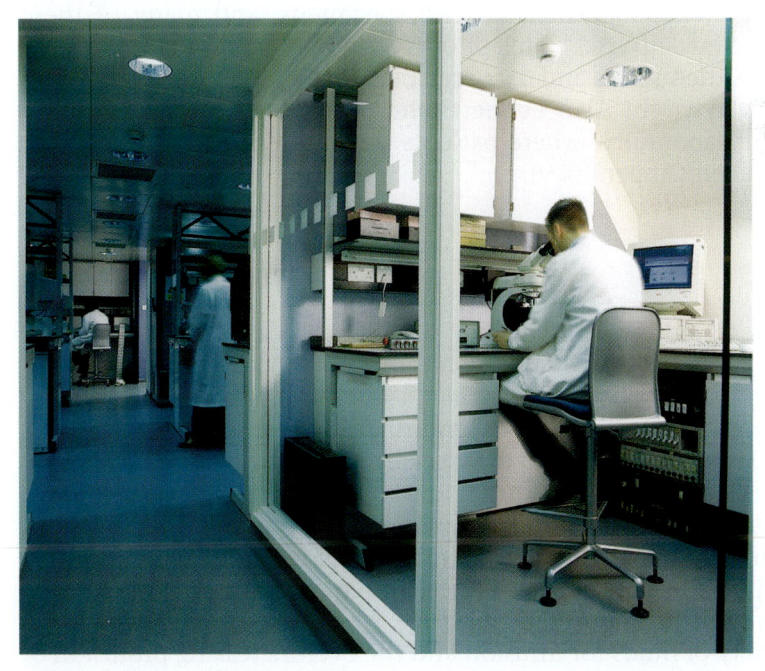

Figure 19.2 *Pathology Department – microscopy equipment.*

Medical Corps, succeeded Dr Tony Chaazan. His interest was in investigating the role of stem cell replacement. In 1990, a unit was established to provide flow cytometry and cryopreservation. This unit had liquid nitrogen storage facilities and was the first of its kind in a private hospital. In 1994, a purpose-built, five-bed, stem cell treatment unit was installed on the second floor.

In October 1995, a case became notorious, when 'Child B', who had been refused treatment by the NHS, was treated at the Clinic. She was given innovative treatment using donor lymphocytes from her sister, which was initially successful and probably extended her life by a year. Since then, transplant work has been expanded at the Clinic, and the work of the department is recognized by the British Society for Bone Marrow Transplantation and was accredited in 2001. This was the first such unit to be given recognition in the private sector. The department is now growing rapidly and is accredited by the European Group of Blood and Bone Marrow Transplantation (EBMT).

A team of biochemical scientists, expert in monitoring autoanalysers, is required to undertake the bulk analyses of inpatients and outpatients attracted to the laboratory. This is now a highly computerized operation, and the results can be downloaded onto clinicians' computers.

Efficient management is required in all modern endeavours, and the laboratory is no exception. Paul Apps leads a team of support staff from his office on the first floor, and results are processed and delivered to clinicians swiftly. More than 2,000 clinicians send specimens, and many of these require results to be delivered by telephone. Specimens are sometimes taken by the clinicians themselves and delivered personally or by courier. In October 2000, the playwright Alan Bennett officially opened the new ground-floor outpatient laboratory, where patients not resident in the Clinic can have samples taken (Appendix 9).

Pharmacy

When I began to study pharmacology as a preclinical student, some 20 years after the Clinic was founded, the number of important drugs in clinical use was modest – probably fewer than a hundred. There were no dressing packs, a limited range of intravenous fluids and only a few drugs scheduled as dangerous and therefore requiring careful failsafe dispensing and administration.

A modest dispensing counter in the basement and limited storage were all that was required – and visiting it was a bit like going into an old-fashioned hardware shop and asking for a padlock, hinge or 100 watt bulb (Figure 19.3). Eventually the unit outgrew the space, which had to house hundreds of drugs, a variety of fluids for infusion and the ever-increasing profusion of antibiotics and chemotherapeutic agents. Storage conditions were difficult

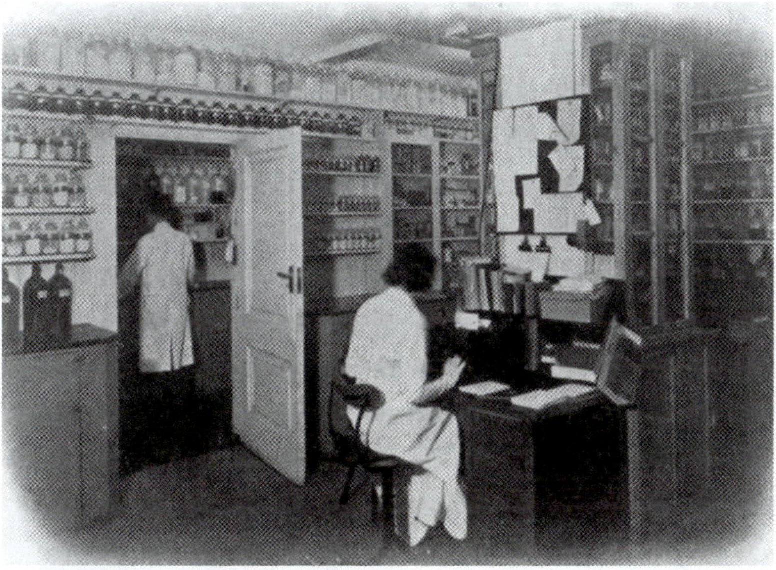

Pathology and pharmacy

Figure 19.3 *Pharmacy in the basement.*

to control and working conditions in the basement less than satisfactory; relocation was inevitable. Gilbert Rees initially started to modernize the department and did such a good job that he was ultimately chosen to be house governor.

The department was brought above ground in the early 1970s and now occupies a prime site off the front hall. A side entrance is used for internal hospital deliveries, and the counter is easily accessible for outpatients (Figure 19.4). Great responsibility is devolved on the staff who provide the service, and now number 20. They dispense, check and monitor prescriptions and have an essential responsibility in helping to prevent human error by prescribers. They flit around the well-lit and airy department, visiting the shelves of drugs, preparing orders from within and without like butterflies and bees in a summer garden. They provide a personal link between the patients and the pills they are dispensing. These have a variety of colours, rivalling an herbaceous border, and are as well known to the staff as are flowers to insects. The patients each leave with a paper bag bearing the Clinic's logo – much like children having visited Father Christmas. Their belief in the medicines is much the same.

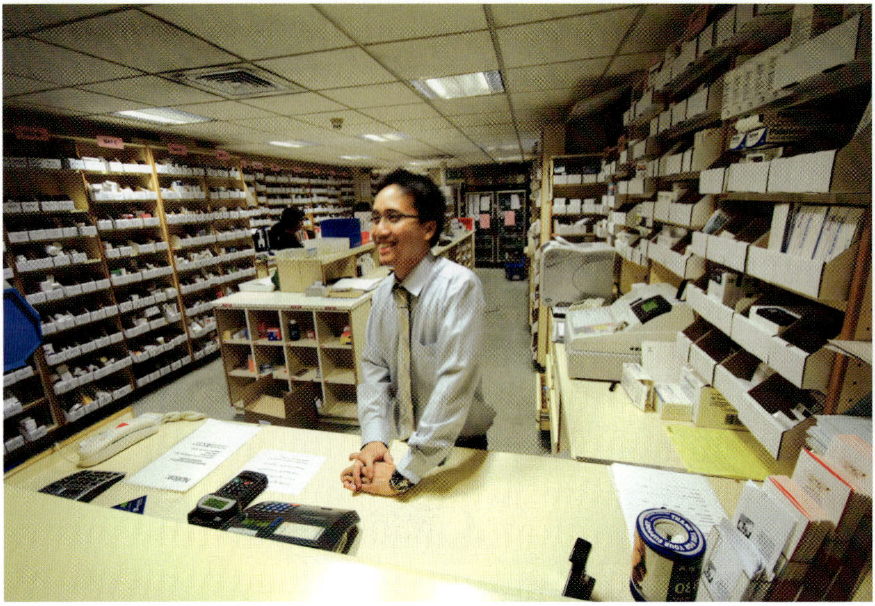

Figure 19.4 *A patient's view of the pharmacy counter today.*

20

Making it happen – house governors and chief executive

Ernest Morris (later Sir Ernest) was the first house governor and ultimately was appointed a governor. When the Clinic went into receivership, he initially resigned, and Mr H Kingsley Pearce, from Leeds General Infirmary, was appointed. His reign was transient, however, and Morris ultimately continued as house governor. Morris had brought Gilbert Rees with him from the London Hospital as his assistant to help organize and equip the Clinic. Rees was initially chief pharmacist and buying officer. During the early part of the war, he was in the Emergency Medical Service. Gilbert Rees succeeded Ernest Morris as house governor and served until his deputy, Michael Jenner, took over (see Appendix 3 for dates).

Dick Kent came from the Royal Marsden Hospital as deputy until he succeeded Jenner. The tradition of the deputy replacing the house governor continued, with Malcolm Miller appointed as such until he took over from Dick Kent. By this time, the post was more appropriately referred to as 'chief executive', in keeping with modern managerial style. The important developments they oversaw and their personal contributions are detailed in the chapters relating to the chairman with whom each worked.

From 1974, clinical activities were regulated under the Nursing Home Act. Since then, further significant changes in regulation procedures have occurred with the Care Standards Act of 2000 and the Health and Social Welfare Act of 2003, which was launched in 2004. As far as the Department of Health is concerned, the Clinic now receives advice via the National Institute of Health and Clinical Excellence (NICE). It is not obligatory to comply, but any recommendations usually are adopted as representing best practice at the time.

As decreed by the Government, the Chief Executive is now legally answerable for the clinical care as well as the administration. The committees which were required to underpin the management of the Clinic – both administrative as well as clinical – have undergone a steady evolution over the years. This was initially dictated by the whims of the Chairman but increased out of all recognition in the nineties and became enshrined in the Health and Social Welfare Act. This dramatic increase was partly the result of the new management style demanded by the times with lines of reporting and formal directorates replacing *ad hoc* committees and personal communication. These are all now co-ordinated by Andrew Barker, Corporate Services Director. He has to be an expert juggler racing from one committee to another and ought to demand special accident insurance as he rushes across the Marylebone Road from his office to the Clinic.

The tiers of committees are shown in Appendices 4 and 5, together with a list of specialty user groups. The requirement for continuing clinical accreditation and professional development has been a catalyst for clinical multidisciplinary committees. These form an important part of life nowadays – not only because they monitor care but also because they bring together the whole care team, including nurses, clinicians, laboratory and diagnostic services. This regular audit is important to ensure that 'best practice' is met and that any deviation from this is not 'swept under the carpet'. The hospital and clinicians have to be able to survive in a very public world of audit that is easily available on the web. In support of these requirements is a large medical records department, which was started originally in 1995. It is now electronic, and confidentiality is strictly regulated in accordance with the Data Protection Act 1998. Kathy Perkins was the first manager. She was also consulting rooms manager in charge of the 149 receptionist staff. They became the first group of staff in the Clinic successfully to undertake NVQs, and the certificates were formally presented to all the candidates by the chairman, Michael Abrahams.

The chairman of the ethics committee, as is proper, is not a clinician and, moreover, is independent from the hospital. The first incumbent, Mr Brian Burgess, a solicitor, chaired the committee from its inception until his death in May 2007. Interestingly enough, one member of the original committee – a tax accountant (John Avery Jones) – is the son of one of our previous distinguished physicians, Sir Francis Avery Jones. It is pleasing that loyalty and belief in the ethos of the Clinic are not only found in patients.

The directorates needed to service the new managerial structure are in keeping with the bureaucracy of our present age. This has been described by the writer Mary McCarthy as the rule of no one, which has become the modern form of despotism! The directorates are listed in Appendix 8, and the number of staff employed approaches 25% of the nursing establishment. This is similar to the ratio found in NHS hospitals; this may well have to be addressed in any future cost savings when administrative techniques improve and globalization and outsourcing by competitors begins to bite.

21
Information technology

The seeds of the information technology (IT) department were sown in the pathology department, and the soil was not barren. It was watered by a report by Peat, Marwick and McLintock in 1990, which, in addition to advising the appointment of a finance director (destined to be Malcolm Miller), also identified the need for an IT department. They rightly realized that this was the only way to manage all the complicated finances, including the vexed question of patient accounts. Mike Worthington in biochemistry and Ron Waite in histology had grasped the early initiative and demonstrated aptitude, competence and amazing foresight by cutting their teeth on the computerized integrated medical laboratory system (CIMLS) and its interface with the finance system (OPTIM). They were able to identify the patient revenue loss and electronically plug the leak. At this time, email was not used and personal computers (PCs) were rare. It was, therefore, a considerable innovation when Medax (a revenue-capturing IT system for private hospitals) was introduced in 1992. Within two or three years of the original report by Peat, Marwick and McLintock, an IT infrastructure was developed and an Apex system installed in the pathology department.

Paper records were still being stored on microfilm by the medical records department. During the late 1990s, however, upon the appointment of Kathy Perkins, the first qualified medical records manager, and in response to the requirements of clinical governance, Medsafe (a document-scanning system) was set up by Ron Waite. With the approval of the Clinic's legal advisers, this was introduced into the medical records department. Therefore, after discharge, patients' records could be safely scanned and stored in a secure system in case of future admission. A fast secure method is now used to enable patients' paper records to be stored electronically and be available for subsequent perusal by appropriate staff and consultants when dealing with any further admissions. Throughout the Clinic, including the nursing floors, are some 600 linked desktop computers. These have to be renewed every five years and therefore represent a considerable but essential financial outlay. The IT structure supports the main Clinic building, the administrative offices in Park Square West and the new consulting rooms in 5 Devonshire Place. Future plans will, of course, have to take in the new cancer centre being developed in Devonshire Place. An extensive interactive website also allows patients to book appointments and treatment online and, indeed, coordinate this with the NHS system. All of these developments, including telemedicine and the patient archiving and communication system (PACS) are being introduced by Mike Roberts, the IT director.

Communications are vital within the Clinic, as well as with the outside world. This is now served by the developing intranet facility, which will greatly assist internal communications and can be used for accessing documents, policies and procedures of the Clinic and indeed other specialist hospitals. The possibility of extending this is being explored in a number of ways and is a further example of the value of IT in the clinical environment.

22

Lest we forget and *The London Clinic Medical Journal*

Hostilities 1914–8, 1939–45 and after

The spirit of the medical profession during wars was characteristically demonstrated by Josephine (later Dame) Barnes, a prominent Harley Street obstetrician, before and after the Clinic had a maternity licence. She continued to undertake domiciliary visits, with two mattresses strapped to the roof of her car to protect her against bomb debris. In September 1939, the two top floors of the Clinic were evacuated and the walls strengthened. Jean Hathorn, who was born in the Clinic in 1934, remembers her physician father, Horace Evans, fire-watching from the roof – as did many other clinicians. Dickson Wright – a prominent surgeon in his own time, who is still remembered as one of the Clinic's great characters – helped to keep the Clinic alive in a variety of ways during these dark days.

The legacy of the Great War (1914–8) and Second World War (1939–45) were borne home recently during excavations for the new cancer centre. Bombs were known to have fallen here in both wars, but happily no unexploded bomb has been found to hinder construction (see Appendix 13).

The operating theatres were moved to the basement – temporarily – and they were destined to return there some 40 years later. Night nurses slept on the sixth floor, and, at night, patients on the third and fourth floors went to the basement, where shelters had been constructed. In September 1940, six houses in Harley Street were destroyed by bombs; the nearest to the Clinic was number 121. Taxis were used as part of the fire service and as many as 2,600 were pressed into service with the Air Raid Precaution (ARP) services. The taxis were used as staff cars and carried explosives for demolishing dangerous buildings (Figure 22.1). I now think back to those days whenever I flag down a cab outside 149.

Skills and expertise were shared around freely at the time and TG Rees, our house governor, advised on equipping base hospitals in three different places. Clinic consultants were involved in surgically changing the facial

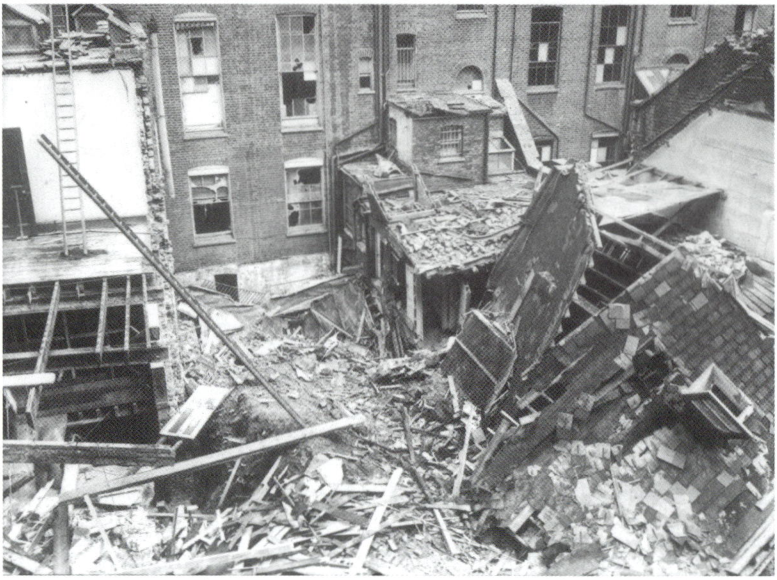

Figure 22.1 *Bomb damage in Marylebone. Reproduced with kind permission from the City of Westminster Archives Centre.*

appearance of some key players in undercover operations with the Special Operating Executive (SOE). Archie Sinclair, the Air Minister, and General Dwight D Eisenhower, Commander-in-Chief of the Second Front, both worked from the Clinic while they were patients.

One of the legendary characters of the war, Odette Hallowes (Figure 22.2), was admitted for treatment after being tortured in Fresnes prison at the hands of her German captors – partly in the mistaken belief that she was related to the prime minister, as her collaborator in the resistance in France

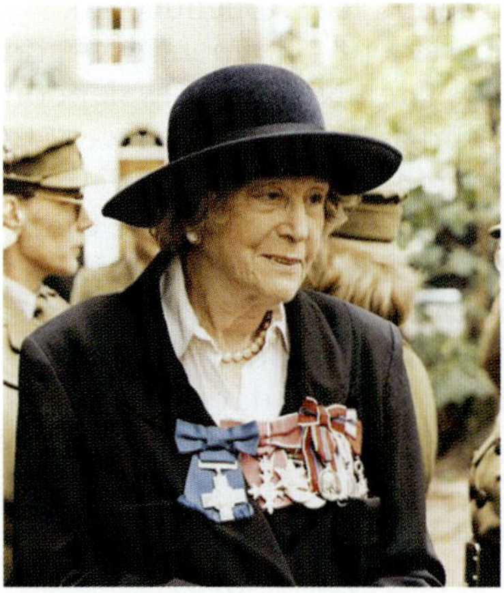

Figure 22.2 *Odette Hallowes GC, MBE, seen wearing her George Cross and Chevalier de Légion d'Honneur. Reproduced with kind permission from the First Aid Nursing Yeomanry (The Princess Royal's Volunteer Corps) (FANY (PRVC)).*

was called Peter Churchill. She was sent to Ravensbrük concentration camp and was the first woman to be awarded the George Cross. She showed great strength of character before weakness, decadence and lack of resolve became more acceptable in modern times as identified recently by Lord Tebbit.

In a later conflict – the Suez Crisis – the Clinic once more played an important role. While Anthony Eden and Major Salem, Egyptian Minister of Propaganda at the time of Suez, metaphorically glared at each other across the canal, they were content to smile at each other when united by the bond of infirmity when in the Clinic.

In more recent times, when stresses between the Turkish and Greek communities in Cyprus came to a head (1959), a Turkish Airline Viscount crash-landed at Gatwick, having been diverted from Heathrow with the Turkish Prime Minister Adnam Menderes on board. Mr Karamanlis, who was representing Greek interests, was also flying into London for the signing of a peace treaty after long negotiations conducted in Zurich. Mr Menderes was taken to the Clinic, and a peace treaty between the Greek and Turkish communities was signed in room 325. Other signatories were Mr Karamanlis, Archbishop Makarios and Prime Minister Kutchuk, with Harold McMillan representing the British government. This gave Cyprus independence but allowed the British to keep a military base on the island. The political situation in Turkey deteriorated, however, and there was a military coup in May 1960. In 1961, Mr Menderes was tried for war crimes against the state and executed.

The London Clinic Medical Journal

I was somewhat surprised when undertaking research on circulating malignant cells as a senior surgical registrar to be referred to an article in the *The London Clinic Medical Journal* by John Griffiths, who was a senior colleague and mentor. The deficiency of a medical library at the Clinic has been mentioned elsewhere; however, the fact that the Clinic once boasted a serious scientific journal often escapes attention (Figure 22.3). Inevitably, the first issue in 1960 also included important in-house pieces, such as the obituary of Sir Harold Gilles. Lord Evans and Sir Aynsley Bridgland wrote an introduction to the first issue.

Such ventures usually were started by enthusiasts, and one must assume that Sir Rodney Maingot (Figure 22.4) was such an enthusiast, as he was chairman of the first editorial committee (1960). After the obituary of the life of Sir Harold Gillies, those of others followed – Conrad Meredyth Hinds Howell (the first to inject the Gasserian ganglion), Lord Evans, Sir Henry Soutar, Dr Ronald Couch, Sir Philip Manson-Barr, Viscount Grantham (chairman of the board of governors [1966–8] and Kathleen, Lady Bridgeland.

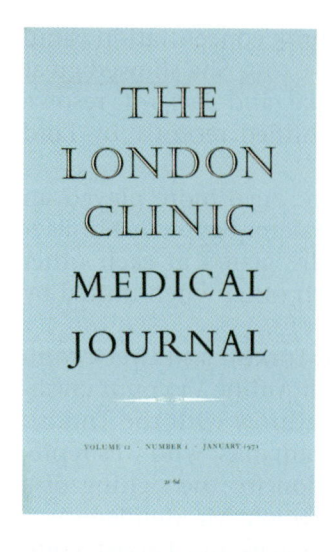

Figure 22.3 *Cover of our Journal.*

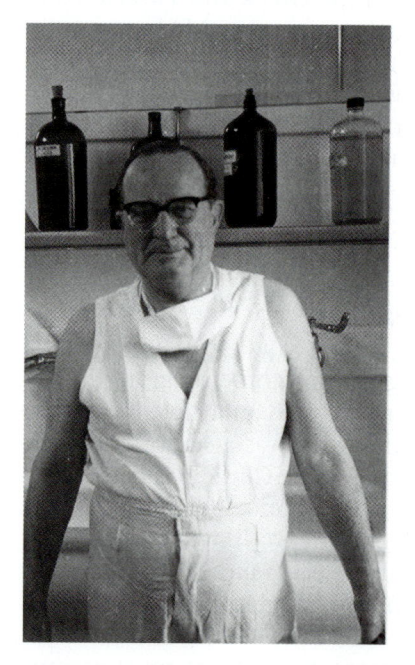

Figure 22.4 *Sir Rodney Maingot.*

By 1970, enthusiasm was flagging. This may have resulted from the need for contributors to publish in international journals and acquire that all-important citation index. The journal, however, fulfilled a need at the time and served to promote the Clinic and the pre-eminence of the staff. It remains an important clinical archive. Appendices 10 and 11 contain the

Lest we forget

tables of contents, which reflect the clinical and other issues of the day. Occasionally clinical update conferences are now held for general practitioners which both educate and inform them of recent developments.

Although the journal is no longer published, communication continues to be important. The Clinic has a website that is constantly updated, a newsletter and a clinical bulletin that keeps general practitioners abreast of new advances and services. A staff news letter, TLC, was published in September 2000 by the inaugural joint editors Kathy Perkins, Paul Apps and Mike Sims; it continues to promote both loyalty and a sense of common purpose and morale. A fledgling staff newsletter, Number Twenty, had been started by Dick Kent, along with George Armson, Ernest Brooksbank, Kathy Brown, Tracey Malcolm, Geraldine Reid and Anna Steven, but soon disappeared as key editors left.

23

Veterans and Christmas

The strength of any institution such as the Clinic is the staff, and this is recognized by a personnel and human resources department. Long service is a happy feature of those employed, with over 50 members of staff serving for more than 20 years, and many more than 30 years. This is especially true of the memorable nursing sisters, who have benignly ruled their domains over the years, humouring the doctors, cherishing the

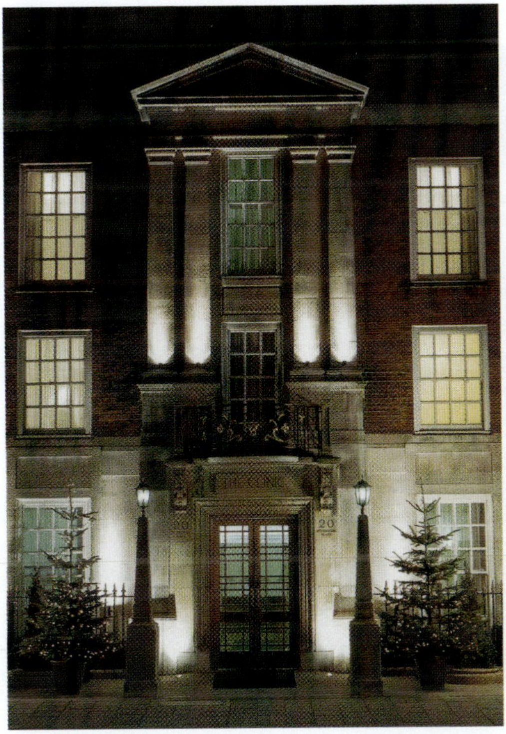

Figure 23.1 *20 Devonshire Place at Christmas.*

patients and watching over the nurses. They are one of our strongest assets. In no way neglected, however, are the technicians, receptionists, porters and all other staff. At the veterans' gatherings once a year, it is possible to rekindle friendships and exchange memories with those like Rene Shingles – who was 35 years in matron's office and would qualify as our universal favourite aunt. Mirroring her in my own life was Sian Turner, my secretary for nearly 30 years. She started in the pathology laboratory aged 18 years and then served as a medical secretary. I was lucky enough to inherit her when my senior colleague in 149, Graham Hayward, died. These are just two isolated examples of loyal service and there are countless others.

None of us is allowed to fade away like an old soldier, but we are all kept in the fold. Loyalty is not an issue, but friendships are renewed between staff of all descriptions. Continuing contact, either personal or via a newsletter, with veterans can be invaluable. Robert Crawford, previously of the Pathology Department was, as a result, able to give us his copies of *The London Clinic Medical Journal*. These are probably the only ones now in existence. At the gatherings we are informed of the changes and planned developments, and after generous hospitality we return home hoping that if ever illness overtakes us in our declining years, we may find a safe haven in the Clinic.

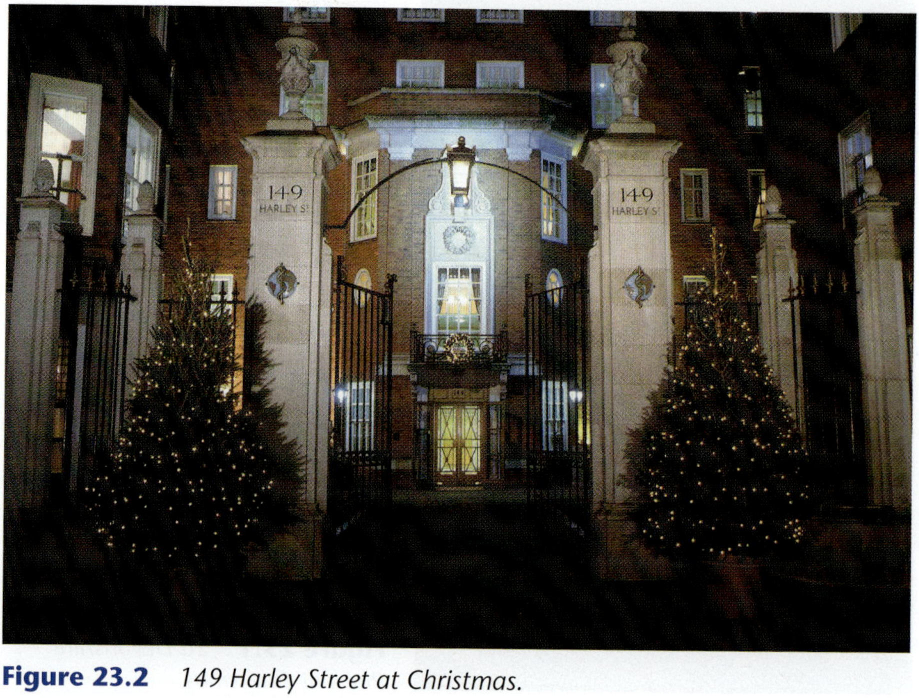

Figure 23.2 *149 Harley Street at Christmas.*

Christmas is always a special time in hospitals, with the consultants touring the wards and keeping alive the traditional generosity that used to be dispensed by our well-to-do Victorian and Edwardian ancestors to dependents and estate workers. This is now directed at the patients. The consultants, in their turn, receive a bonus from some satisfied patients in the form of hampers from Fortnum and Mason, which are wheeled to their consulting rooms on a porter's trolley. The governors also generously recognize, with the gift of a hamper, those who have served on committees. I was always relieved not to see a clandestine tax inspector listing the benefits in kind that were being received in the consulting rooms. All of these festivities culminate in the lavish Christmas reception arranged by the governors for the staff and visiting consultants. The Christmas reception for the nurses in 1945 cost £116 and a ball at the Savoy Hotel in 1949 just £114.2.4d. Fortunately, our enjoyment of the Christmas reception is not spoiled by knowing its cost, which although it must be considerable, is a good investment in loyalty and appreciation. There is much fun, food and music at the generous reception given by the governors, which in recent years has been held at the Royal Academy of Music. On an occasion like this, we all realize how much the Clinic means to the staff. The singing of carols and donations to Christmas charities helps to repay our debt to society.

24

We have lift off

We live in an age when the ability to reach one planet leads to the targeting of another. The quest is never-ending, like the frontiers of medicine, where nothing stands still. One accomplishment, even in space, leads logically to another challenge. The Clinic has to keep change and expectations always in its sights. Its own space is unhappily constrained by its position and the limitation of the planners; however, clever strategic planning means that changes wrought within the building have enabled an impressive range of services to be provided on site.

Outposts have been developed in Harley Street – at numbers 114–118, 119, 145 and 147. New state-of-the-art consulting rooms at 5 Devonshire Place – the old headquarters of the Medical Defence Union – were officially opened on 6 February 2007 by the Duchess of Devonshire as part of the multi-site development programme known as Project Quantum Leap. This building houses 25 custom-designed consulting suites (Figure 24.1), which will enable some 50 consultants to vacate number 149, which can then, in turn, be incorporated into the main clinical building to give valuable extra space and also provide a more appropriate entrance to the Clinic from Harley Street. Many outpatient services are located in the new consulting rooms, of which the largest is diabetic screening. Ultrasound, x-ray, echocardiography, lung function, bone densitometry, colposcopy and endocrinology all feature prominently. This is convenient for the patients and more efficient for the medical staff.

The 'big bang' of Project Quantum Leap will be the development of the most up-to-date comprehensive cancer unit across Devonshire Place, linked to the main building by an underground tunnel. This will house consulting suites, chemotherapy and radiotherapy units. The site has been cleared, and the opening is planned for the summer of 2009. Acquisition of the site required complicated negotiations with five different owners and leaseholders. Some held out with varying degrees of determination, but acceptable terms ultimately were agreed, allowing the project to start (see Appenices 13 and 14).

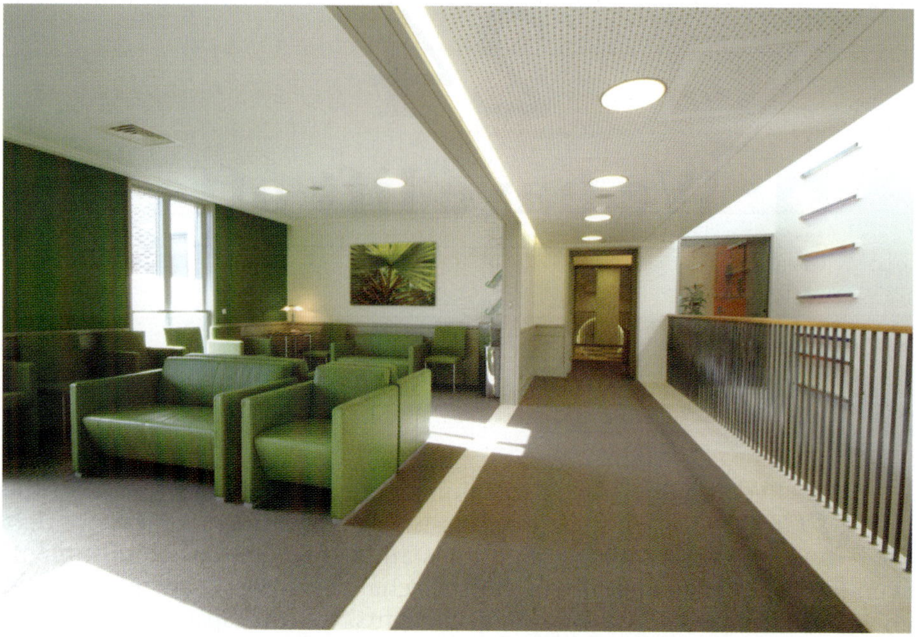

Figure 24.1 *A waiting room in the new outpatient building 5 Devonshire Place – the doctors consulting rooms have a more individual but not dissimilar decor.*

This development is, in many ways, the product of clinical need. Cancer patients have always been drawn to the Clinic to be looked after by physicians and surgeons with a specialist interest. Dr Peter Wrigley (who had been senior registrar to Professor Gordon Hamilton Fairley, who died as a result of a bomb planted by the Irish Republican Army) had an interest in the developing field of chemotherapy. He worked in conjunction with surgeons at the Clinic both from general hospitals and the Royal Marsden Hospital – a specialist cancer hospital. A cohort of younger physicians expert in the rapidly developing field of medical oncology focussed their skills on the Clinic. Leader of these was Dr Maurice Slevin, who had, early in his clinical career, been a founding force in Cancerbackup. He was the catalyst and driving force in the exponential growth of the oncology unit and was supported by Dr Peter Harper and the late Dr David Gueret Wardle. The future importance of oncology is ensured, as demonstrated and confirmed by the development of the new cancer centre.

None of these developments would have been possible and, indeed, could not have been contemplated without the Clinic being a financially secure charity that returned all of its profits for the future benefit of patients. These ambitious developments are a fine memorial to Sir Aynsley Bridgland and will be a lasting tribute to the efficient and inspired management of the trustees. This has been possible because of the remarkable clinical expertise that it has attracted and the abiding loyalty of staff and patients who have passed through the doors.

In clinical care, a relentless march from the general to the particular is taking place. This has been driven partly by evidence-based medicine and technology but also by audit, information sharing and now the benefits of continuing professional development. The Clinic first addressed this trend by having specialist nursing floors (see page 67) and ensuring that nursing education played an important part in the process. Once these skills were in place, specialists were happy to entrust their patients to the Clinic. The consultants who practice in many of the specialist areas are now bound together in 'specialist user groups' (see Appendix 5), and the patients are audited in regular meetings – the multidisciplinary committees. In addition to specialist nurses, many of the new disciplines require special diagnostic equipment (e.g. for mammography and exercise cardiography) or special treatment areas and aftercare facilities (e.g. for oncology).

Over the years, continuity of medical care between consultants' visits has been provided by resident medical officers, often those studying for exams or awaiting appointment in the NHS. Recently, postgraduate doctors have come to maintain clinical experience while undertaking research degrees. This scheme was negotiated with Professor Marc Winslet at the Royal Free Hospital.

The degree of care and supervision that patients in specialist units require demands more than the traditional support from a general resident medical officer. Most of the dedicated clinical groups have their own clinical fellows in training, who look after the patients in that particular specialty. These are almost invariably funded by the Clinic. They can, however, call in other expertise if necessary, such as the in-house cardiac emergency team.

The units are at varying stages of development, the oncology unit being one of the oldest (and largest) and the liver unit, under its director Professor Roger Williams, internationally recognized but only recently having taken rooms at the Clinic, the youngest.

None of these developments could have come to pass without the injection of capital together with administrative and clinical enthusiasm. The education of nurses in these specialist fields, however, has been paramount. As in everything medical, a good team spirit is of the greatest importance. Those three guiding lights in clinical training of which we must never lose sight are apprentices, mentors and heroes.

Box 24.1 summarizes the main clinical specialties that are now provided and Box 24.2 their diagnostic and support services. Chemotherapy and stem cell harvesting (in conjunction with the Anthony Nolan Trust and Bone and Marrow Transplantation) are undertaken as daycare or short-term inpatient procedures. In addition to the ethically approved research undertaken by consultants wholly at the Clinic or in conjunction with their NHS hospitals, there are training placements for 30 nursing, 20 radiological and

Box 24.1   *Current main clinical specialties.*
- Allergy
- Breast surgery
- Cardiology
- Dermatology
- Diabetes
- Ear, nose and throat (ENT)
- Endocrinology and endocrine surgery
- Gastroenterology and endoscopy
- Gastrointestinal and colorectal surgery
- General medicine
- General practice
- General surgery
- Genetics
- Genito-urinary medicine
- Gynaecology
- Haematology
- Hepato-biliary services
- Intensive care medicine
- Nephrology/renal and transplant surgery
- Neurology and neurosurgery
- Oncology (including chemotherapy and palliative care)
- Ophthalmology
- Oral and maxillofacial surgery
- Orthopaedics (including specialist spinal and hand)
- Paediatrics
- Pain management
- Plastic and reconstructive surgery (including cosmetic)
- Respiratory medicine
- Rheumatology
- Thoracic surgery
- Urology and nephrology (including lithotripsy)
- Vascular medicine

six physiotherapy students. Also available in the Clinic precincts are Macmillan nurse and Cancerbackup services.

> **Box 24.2** *Diagnostic and support services for current main clinical specialties.*
> - Assessment (cardiopulmonary exercise testing) before surgery
> - Cancerbackup
> - Cardiology
> - Critical care
> - Dialysis
> - Dietetics
> - Endoscopy
> - Gastrointestinal clinical investigation
> - Health screening (including osteoporosis screening)
> - Macmillan nurse service
> - Mammography
> - Mole mapping
> - Neurophysiology
> - Pathology
> - Personal fitness assessment
> - Pharmacy
> - Physiotherapy (including sports injuries and hydrotherapy unit)
> - Radiology and scanning screening (including X-ray, MRI, CT, bone densitometry and ultrasound)
> - Sleep studies

These clinical services are supported at present by 144 inpatient beds and 58 daycare beds. There are 12 operating theatres, three endoscopy theatres and a minimally invasive day surgery unit. As the range of clinical procedures changed there had to be accommodation for chemotherapy, stem cell and bone marrow transplantation as well. This was done in conjunction with the Anthony Nolan Trust.

The Clinic has always attracted charitable donations. Patients and their relatives have, on occasion, either made donations to research projects or, as in the case of The Mary Obolensky Underwood Foundation (MOUF), supported research more formally. In the early days, Bernard Sunley contributed regularly to the Samaritan Fund, and the Clinic in its turn has dispersed funds not only as a charitable discount but also for specific reasons such as the Jubilee Fund (see Appendix 6). Charitable discounts in 2005 amounted to £807,000 for needy patients. In 2006, nearly 8,000 patients were admitted and more than 12,000 day cases, with 63,000 patients attending for outpatient procedures. The vast majority of these patients were residents of the UK.

Efficient use of the facilities in a comparatively small space now enables us to operate at a profit. The fairytale has come true over the past 25 years and enables a large investment in the facilities and equipment. Charities have be accountable and transparent and also run like blue chip companies. Administrators may now be rewarded more generously then many of the specialists who attract patients. They can no longer be allowed the luxury of doing good for its own sake and have to be recruited from a competitive market place.

Banks, among other organizations, attract criticism for their charges and the profit they make – and with some justification. When our statistical profile over the last 15 years is examined, there has been an increase in bed numbers of towards 20% and in specialists with admitting rights of 500%. There are 145 consultants and these are accommodated in 90 consulting suites – there having been no more than 35 consultants for many years. The operating surplus generated has risen by a factor of four times the increase in the number of specialists and the net assets have had an even greater exponential rise. The justification for being such a successful business is that, unlike the banks, the profits are all used to improve and expand clinical services, thus fulfilling the charitable status. It is likely – and perhaps desirable – that the rate of growth and operating surplus will plateau somewhat after the cancer centre opens. This will allow consolidation before consideration of how the Clinic can spread its expertise, experience and ethos more widely.

Although one can applaud the success, one wonders how much longer patients in this country will tolerate the stress of travel, parking and personal security in the inner city to seek expertise – especially as centres of excellence are distributed more uniformly than they were a few years ago. In America, this has been solved by moving private hospitals to the peripheries of large cities and having regional satellites. This may well have to be addressed in this country. There is also the possibility of telemedicine – already explored by the Clinic a few years ago. The future remains a challenge to which I am sure the Clinic with its new dynamism will respond.

The institution is, of course, larger than the sum of the constituent parts, and the ethos of the Clinic and the welfare of the patients is the gold standard for the future.

All this shows the total commitment to all aspects of medicine, including research, training and education. All the strategic planning and challenges would come to little without the continuing loyalty of the staff – clinical and others – who work as a team and have a commitment to the institution.

May the present morale be maintained to secure the future.

Appendices

Appendices

1
Acknowledgements listing

It has been a pleasure to have been associated with all of those involved with the book. Most of them are listed below.

Interviews and written submission papers

Abrahams, Michael
Anyan, Frank
Apps, Paul
Baldwin, Jane
Baldwin, Steve
Barker, Andrew
Barton, Peter
Beecroft, Tony
Boden, Betty
Booth, John Barton (late) and son James
Bowden, Richard (Howard de Walden Archivist)
Brooksbank, Ernest
Bullivant, Karen
Capital Planning and Works Departments, The London Clinic
Colman, Cynthia
Dick, Robert
Duchess of Devonshire, The
Dutton, Sylvia
Dyer, Chris
Edgcombe, Chris
Ferrand, Gillian
Francis-Saati, Pierre Maher
Garfield Davies, David
Garratt, Dianne
George, Patricia
Geraint James, David
Gerolemou, John
Goodbun, Kevin
Gordon, Carmel
Gorecki, Wanda
Hallums, Amanda
Hathorn, Jean
Henderson, Laura
Hennessey, Peggy
Heyland, Charmian
Holmes Sellors, Patrick
Husband, Janet
Irvine, Gillian
IT department, The London Clinic
Jenner, Michael
Jennings, Mike
Keeler, Ann
Kent, Richard (Dick)
Kirkham, John Squire

Knight, John
Knox, Ken
Local Studies Library, Leeds City Council
Major, Maxine
Marketing department, The London Clinic
Marylebone Public Library
Miller, Malcolm
Morson, Basil
Murray, Val
Neyt, Leigh-Anne
Pearce, Hilary
Pennie, Allan
Peppitt, Andrew (Chatsworth Archivist)
Peters, Bill
Petrou, Sandra
Puzzutti, Christine Dr (Granddaughter of Aynsley Bridgland)
Ramsden, James
Rees, HB
Roberts, Mike
Root, Frank
Rose, Liz
Ross, Harvey
Seear, Tiba
Shah, Sanjay
Shingles, Renee
Sims, Mike
Smyth, Ethna
Stanbury, Anthony
Steven, Anna
Talbot, Ian
Teesdale, James
Tinker, Jack
Trott, Peter
Waite, Ron
Wessely, Hannah
Westminster City Archives Centre
Williams, Christopher B
Williams, JP
Witt (late), Margaret and her sister, Lorna Bartlet
Wood, Paul

2
Clinic mission and philosophy

Operating as an independent, charitable hospital, we dedicate our skills, energies and resources to be the hospital of first choice for patients, specialists and staff. Fully committed to clinical excellence, we aim to exceed our patients' expectations by embracing the very best aspects of traditional patient care, delivered by highly trained staff adopting best clinical practice and using the latest medical technology.

- To undertake initiatives that will reinforce The London Clinic's standing as a successful charitable hospital at the forefront of independent healthcare.
- To excel in every aspect of patient care and to strive for clinical excellence.
- To act at all times with integrity and with respect for the needs of our patients, specialists and staff.
- To value The London Clinic's heritage of delivering traditional patient care while embracing the very best elements of modern medicine.
- To attract and retain highly skilled members of staff by providing support and resources to enable them to carry out their duties effectively, efficiently and with pride.

Our charitable status

As a not-for-profit organization, The London Clinic is able continuously to invest in the latest medical technology, facilities and clinical and nursing support.

As the Clinic does not have any shareholders, in the last five years alone it has been able to invest £64m in improved medical equipment and hospital facilities. This means that, unlike many independent hospitals, the Clinic is able to treat patients with very complex conditions such as brain tumours and liver disorders.

Accreditation

To ensure that The London Clinic's high standards of quality are continuously maintained, rigorous clinical audits are carried out both internally and externally by national regulatory bodies.

3

Chairmen, house governors, chief executive and matrons

Chairmen

8th Duke of Atholl	1932–1935
Sir Aynsley Bridgland	1935–1966
Vincent Alpe Grantham	1966–1968
Sir Tom Hickinbotham	1968–1978
6th Earl of Ranfurly	1978–1984
The Right Honourable James Ramsden	1984–1996
Michael Abrahams	1996–

House governors and chief executive

H Kingsley Pearce	1932–1932
Sir Ernest Morris	1932–1941
Trevor Gilbert Rees	1941–1973
Michael Jenner	1973–1981
Richard (Dick) Kent	1981–1994
Malcolm Miller	1994–

Matrons

Miss M Hebdon	1932–1932
Miss Pinnell	1932–*
Miss M Reynolds	*–1938
Miss Jean D Jacomb	1938–1949

* records deficient

Miss V Joan Lewis	1949–1967
Miss Sylvia Dutton	1967–1979
Miss Laura Henderson	1979–1984
Miss Betty Boden	1984–2003
Miss Amanda Hallums	2003–

4

Governors and trustees, operations board and executive board

Governors and trustees

Mr Michael D Abrahams CBE, DL (chairman)
The Duchess of Devonshire
Mr Richard A Hambro
Sir Christopher Paine DM, FRCR, FRCP
Mr Rupert S Ponsonby
Lady Eccles of Moulton
*Malcolm Miller (chief executive)
*Andrew Barker (corporate services director)
*Tony Beecroft (capital planning director)
*Karen Bullivant (marketing director)
*Amanda Hallums (matron/director of clinical services)
*Gillian Irvine (human resources and training director)
*Mike Roberts (IT director)
*Sanjay Shah (chief financial officer)
*Paul Wood (strategy director)

*In attendance only.

Operations board

Malcolm Miller (chairman)
Andrew Barker
Amanda Hallums
Gillian Irvine
Sanjay Shah

Executive board

Malcolm Miller (chairman)
Andrew Barker
Tony Beecroft
Karen Bullivant
Amanda Hallums
Gillian Irvine
Mike Roberts
Sanjay Shah
Paul Wood

5

Medical advisory committee, chairmen of the medical advisory committee and specialty user groups, 2007

Medical advisory committee

Mr MD Abrahams CBE, DL (chairman)
Dr I Murray-Lyon (medical chairman)
Mr F Afshar
Dr P Amoroso
Professor M Besser
Mr J Brazier
Mr G Brookes
Professor J Cobb
Dr P Ettlinger
Dr P Fairclough
Dr J Goldstone
Professor Dame J Husband
Dr W Marshall
Professor RJ Nicholls
Mr D Ross
Professor J Shepherd
Dr M Slevin
Mr S St Clair Carter
*Mr MP Miller
*Miss A Hallums
*Mr S Shah
*Mr A Barker (Secretary)

*In attendance only.

Medical advisory committee chairmen

Sir Anthony Dawson 1991–1997
Mr John Squire Kirkham 1997–2000
Mr Christopher Russell 2000–2004
Dr Iain Murray-Lyon 2004–

Specialty user groups

Bariatric medicine
Endoscopy
Ear, nose and throat; oral and maxillofacial
General surgical/third floor
General practitioners
Gynaecological
Intensive therapy unit/progressive care unit/Anaesthetics
Minimally invasive treatment unit/daycare surgery unit
Neurology
Oncology
Ophthalmology
Orthopaedics
Physicians
Plastic and reconstructive surgery
Theatre
Urology/nephrology
Vascular

6
Charitable status

The London Clinic is one of the UK's largest and oldest charitable hospitals. It has long had an international reputation for clinical excellence.

The charitable status it enjoys allows every penny of its surplus to be reinvested back into the hospital, continuously allowing facilities and patient care services to be updated. As well as attracting London's leading consultants, the Clinic is respected for the outstanding quality of its personal care of patients.

Information on all aspects of cancer is available to patients and their families. A Cancerbackup information service is located in and funded by the Clinic. This is available free-of-charge to those, whether patients or otherwise, who seek information on cancer and related issues.

A Macmillan nurse is similarly funded and on hand to provide emotional and clinical support to patients with cancer. There is also a separate free oncology counselling service. Most patients with cancer who are treated make use of these services. Complementary therapies such as reflexology and massage are also available free-of-charge.

We are the only independent hospital to provide bone marrow collection, stem cell collection and a harvesting centre for the Anthony Nolan Trust. The medical staff are able to use our state-of-the-art facilities to support the Anthony Nolan Trust in providing donors for patients in need of transplants. Last year we collected approximately 250 donations.

Charitable and humanitarian discounts are provided. During 2005, such discounts approached £1m for various needy patients. The Clinic has recently commenced treating, at a special discount, armed forces personnel referred from another charitable hospital when they are unable to offer all the necessary facilities.

Our charitable status places us in a unique position to advance clinical standards. For example, the Clinic is developing a world-class liver centre for the treatment and diagnosis of liver disease. Next year, we expect to be undertaking liver transplants. A specialist liver research nurse has been appointed and research into the efficacy of new treatments has commenced.

We are able to carry out robotic surgical procedures, most notably for prostatic disease. This allows highly complex and technologically advanced surgical techniques to be undertaken. These are revolutionizing surgery and the patients' recovery.

A fully equipped clinical skills laboratory is available for staff training. The courses are also open to healthcare staff from the NHS and other hospitals on a cost-recovery basis. The Clinic works in partnership with other charities, funding nurses to provide practical support and make available up to 100 clinical placements per year free-of-charge for NHS students. Training is also provided for a plastic surgical fellow awaiting a consultant post within the NHS. Currently, the NHS does not offer this training. We also provide paid placements to 14 doctors below consultant level to support the research period of their training.

We are in the process of establishing a postgraduate medical faculty offering subsidized places to doctors who are undertaking postgraduate medical training before their final examinations to become a Member of the Royal College of Surgeons (MRCS) or Member of the Royal College of Physicians (MRCP). Both NHS and overseas doctors will participate.

Research is undertaken in the Clinic, which advances the science of medicine, involving clinical trials across a large number of specialities. In addition, the charitable status has allowed us to develop expertise in new technologies and treatments that have gone on to have general application elsewhere. An example relates to the development of endoscopic procedures in which advanced techniques have been developed and are now the established form of treatment elsewhere.

Recently we supported a number of important initiatives designed to improve patient care. Our cardiopulmonary exercise testing programme (CPX) is the first in the UK and makes available extensive data which aid the assessment of patients undergoing major surgery. This should significantly improve care, leading to fewer and shorter critical-care admissions. The Clinic is developing a pioneering thrombosis service, which will reduce post-surgical complications, treatment costs and improve patient care.

Many important educational and teaching activities have resulted from practices at the Clinic. Examples include the use of photodynamic therapy and endoscopic ultrasound-guided fine needle aspiration and biopsy.

Last year, we treated more than 90,000 patients who would otherwise have required NHS treatment. Unlike many independent hospitals, the Clinic is able to provide Level 2 and Level 3 critical care with the highest quality of acute intensive care facilities on hand. This avoids patients being transferred out to the NHS if their condition deteriorates. Critical care back-up is also available to other independent hospitals in London. We deliver dialysis treatment as an alternative to the NHS. The Clinic also provides

Appendix 6: Charitable status

state-of-the art chemotherapy and cancer care. We have a large range of scanning services, thus relieving the severe pressure that exists for those services in the NHS.

On the 60th anniversary of The London Clinic in 1992, the trustees initiated an appeal to a broad range of potential donors to establish a fund aimed at providing free treatment to a limited number of patients each year. These had to be permanently resident in London, not covered by private medical insurance and be suffering from conditions that impaired lifestyle. The trustees decided to close this fund in 2003 and transfer the remaining monies to a new fund for staff training and education. A clinical and nursing staff training fund established in 1997 from the proceeds of an exceptional value added tax (VAT) refund had been used for retention and training of nurses and clinical staff. This has since 1997 been invested in Charifunds (M & G Securities).

7
The London Clinic: committee structure

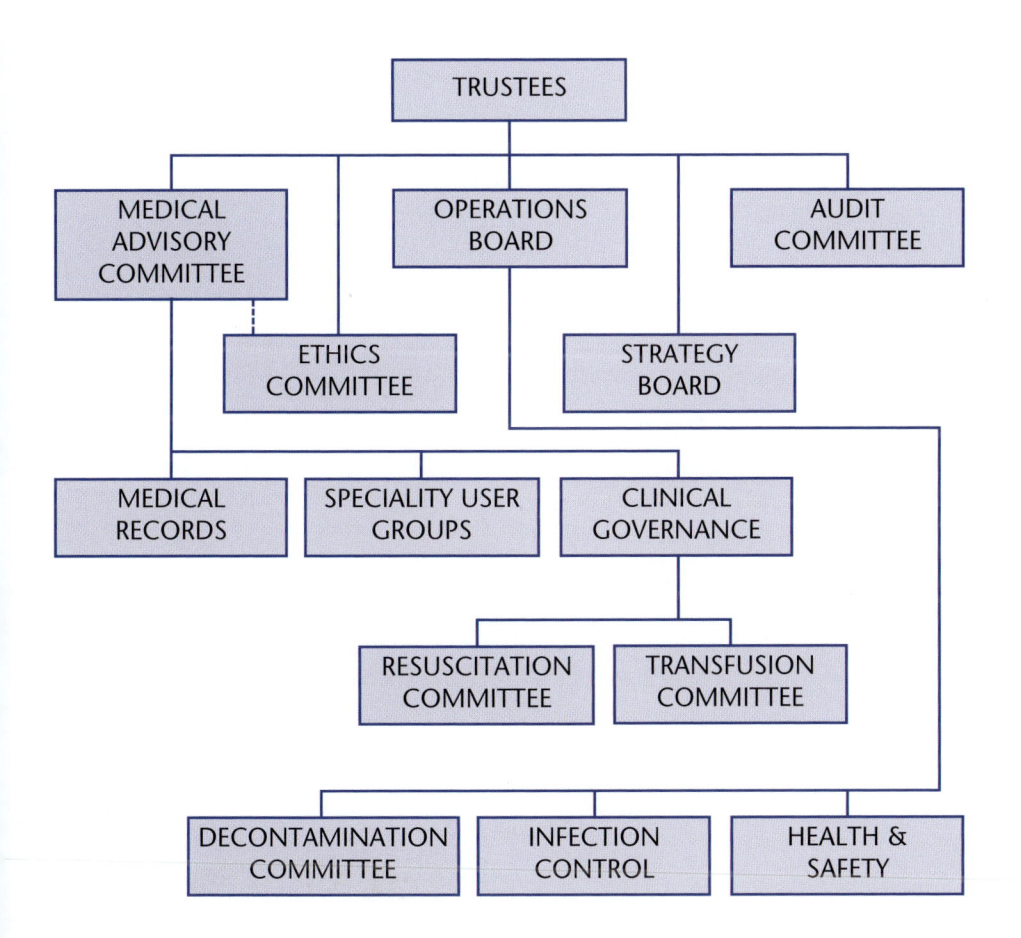

```
                          TRUSTEES
         ┌──────────────────┼──────────────────┐
    MEDICAL            OPERATIONS           AUDIT
    ADVISORY             BOARD           COMMITTEE
   COMMITTEE
        │                   │
      ETHICS            STRATEGY
    COMMITTEE            BOARD

   MEDICAL      SPECIALITY USER     CLINICAL
   RECORDS        GROUPS          GOVERNANCE
                              ┌───────┴───────┐
                         RESUSCITATION    TRANSFUSION
                          COMMITTEE       COMMITTEE

     DECONTAMINATION    INFECTION      HEALTH &
       COMMITTEE         CONTROL        SAFETY
```

7

The London Clinic:
committee structure

8

The London Clinic: organizational charts

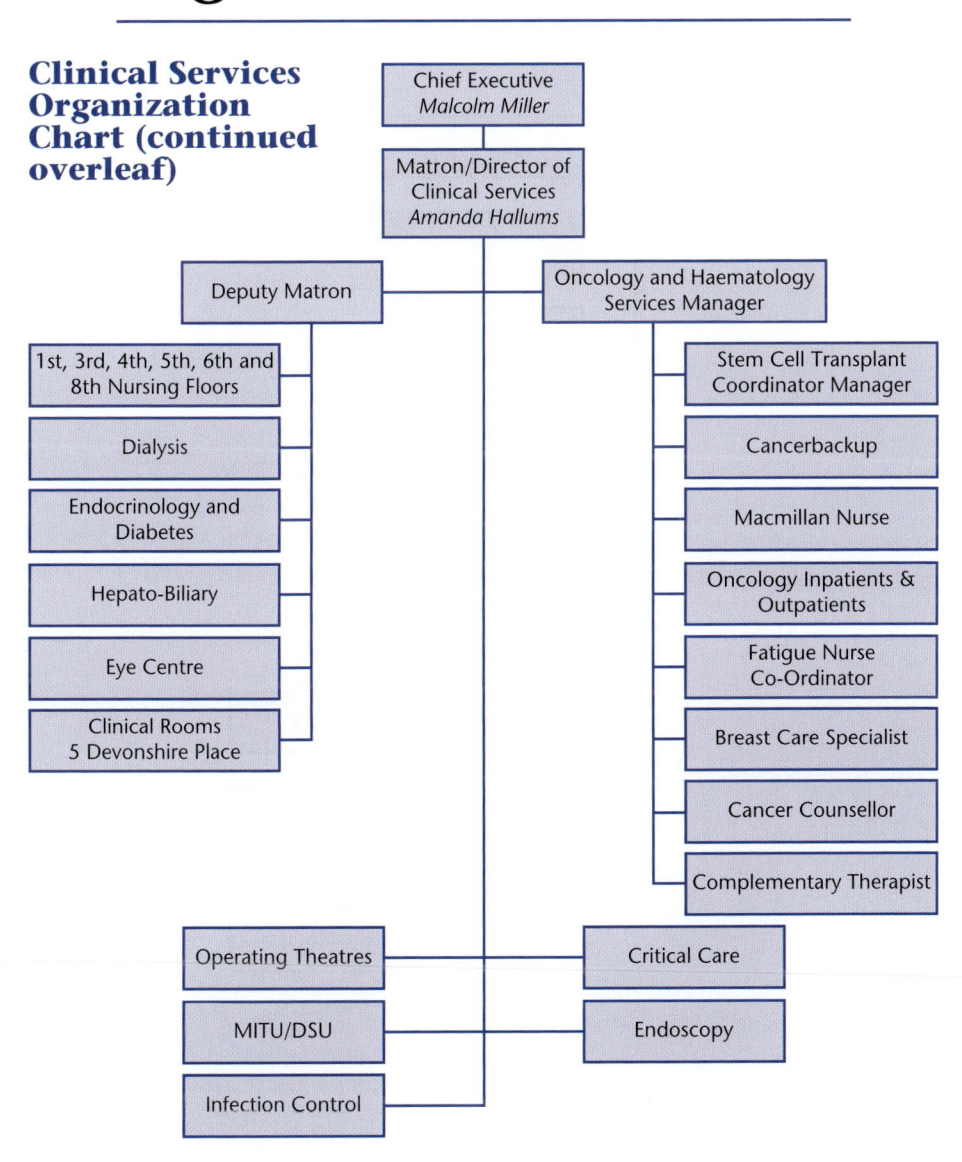

Clinical Services Organization Chart (continued overleaf)

- Chief Executive
  Malcolm Miller
- Matron/Director of Clinical Services
  Amanda Hallums

- Deputy Matron
  - 1st, 3rd, 4th, 5th, 6th and 8th Nursing Floors
  - Dialysis
  - Endocrinology and Diabetes
  - Hepato-Biliary
  - Eye Centre
  - Clinical Rooms 5 Devonshire Place

- Oncology and Haematology Services Manager
  - Stem Cell Transplant Coordinator Manager
  - Cancerbackup
  - Macmillan Nurse
  - Oncology Inpatients & Outpatients
  - Fatigue Nurse Co-Ordinator
  - Breast Care Specialist
  - Cancer Counsellor
  - Complementary Therapist

- Operating Theatres
- MITU/DSU
- Infection Control
- Critical Care
- Endoscopy

Clinical Services Organizational Chart (continued)

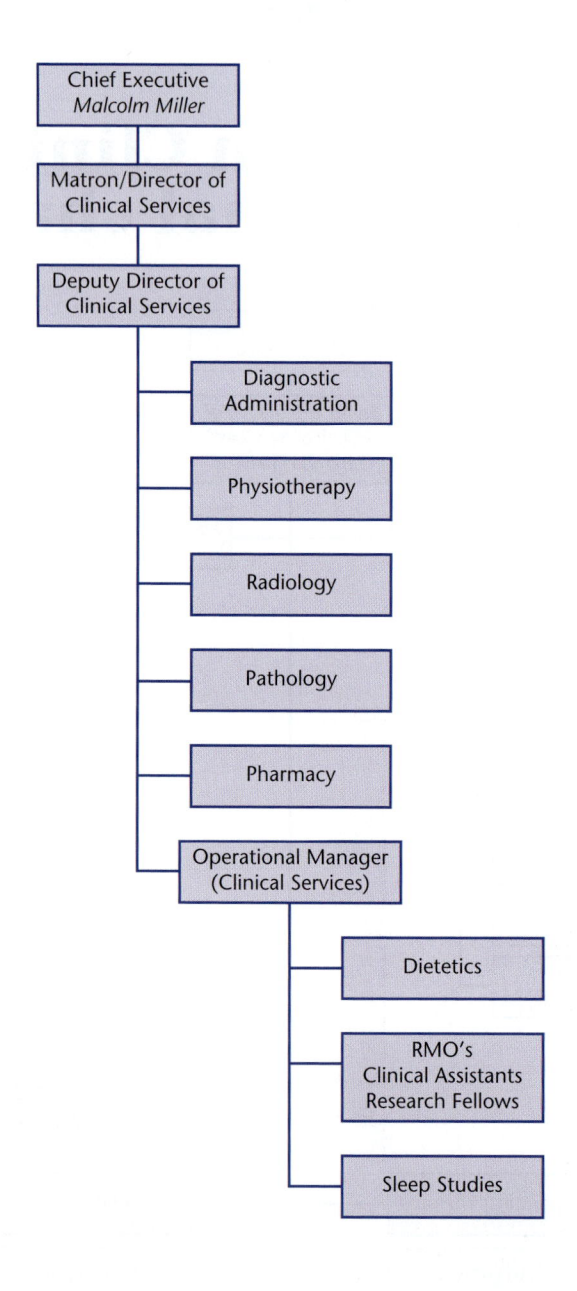

- Chief Executive
  Malcolm Miller
  - Matron/Director of Clinical Services
    - Deputy Director of Clinical Services
      - Diagnostic Administration
      - Physiotherapy
      - Radiology
      - Pathology
      - Pharmacy
      - Operational Manager (Clinical Services)
        - Dietetics
        - RMO's
          Clinical Assistants
          Research Fellows
        - Sleep Studies

Appendix 8: The London Clinic: organizational chart **163**

Non-clinical Services Organization Chart

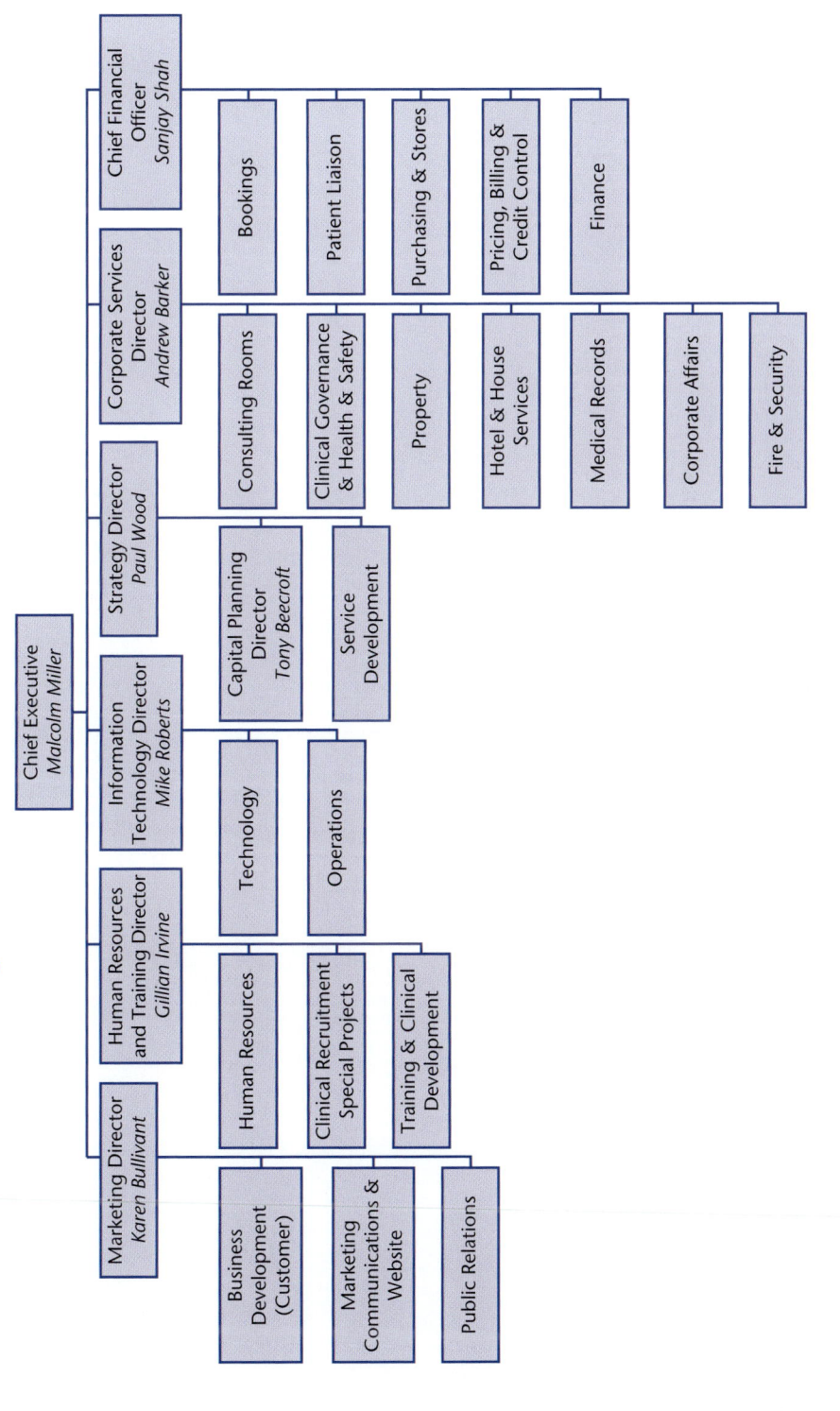

Chief Executive — *Malcolm Miller*

- **Marketing Director** — *Karen Bullivant*
  - Business Development (Customer)
  - Marketing Communications & Website
  - Public Relations

- **Human Resources and Training Director** — *Gillian Irvine*
  - Human Resources
  - Clinical Recruitment Special Projects
  - Training & Clinical Development

- **Information Technology Director** — *Mike Roberts*
  - Technology
  - Operations

- **Strategy Director** — *Paul Wood*
  - Capital Planning Director — *Tony Beecroft*
  - Service Development

- **Corporate Services Director** — *Andrew Barker*
  - Consulting Rooms
  - Clinical Governance & Health & Safety
  - Property
  - Hotel & House Services
  - Medical Records
  - Corporate Affairs
  - Fire & Security

- **Chief Financial Officer** — *Sanjay Shah*
  - Bookings
  - Patient Liaison
  - Purchasing & Stores
  - Pricing, Billing & Credit Control
  - Finance

9
Celebrity openings of departments

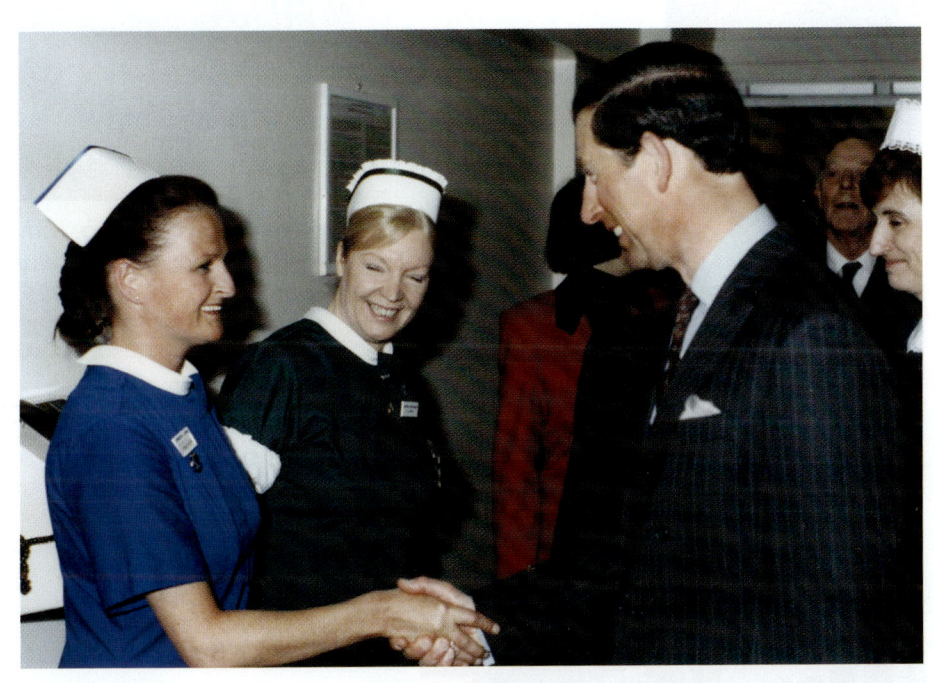

Figure A9.1 *HRH The Prince of Wales, Physiotherapy Department, 1989.*

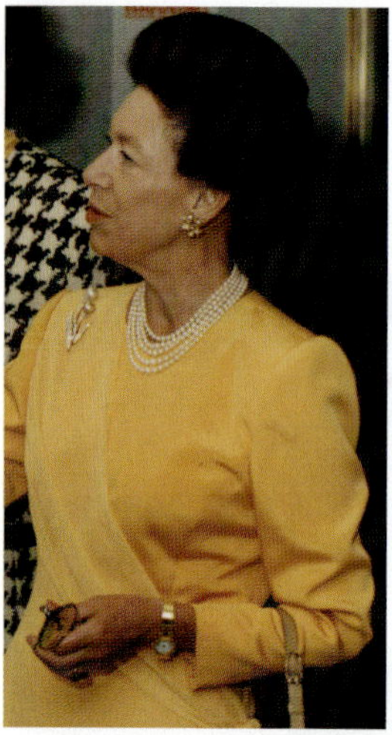

Figure A9.2 HRH The Princess Margaret, magnetic resonance imaging department, 15 October 1991.

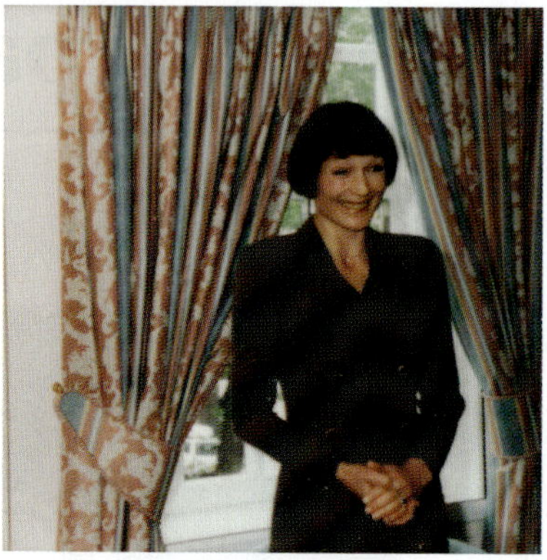

Figure A9.3 Victoria, Lady Getty, minimally invasive therapy unit (MITU), 23 May 1995.

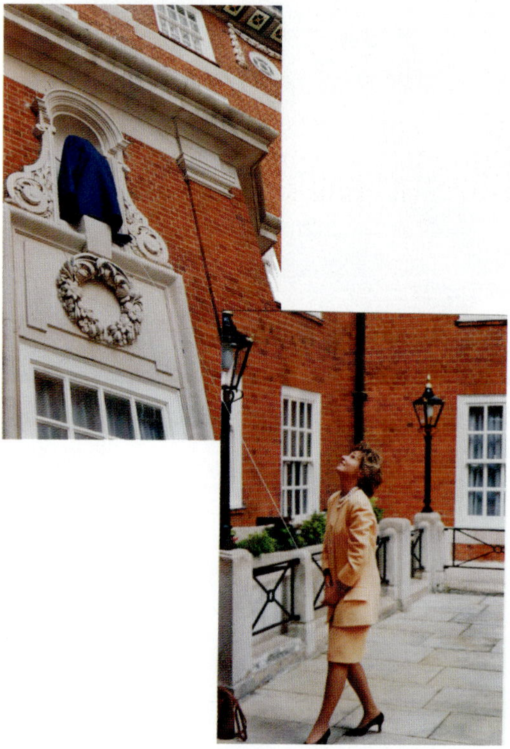

Figure A9.4 Lady Hartington, now Duchess of Devonshire, unveiling the Lady Bacon sculpture, 149 Harley Street, July 1996.

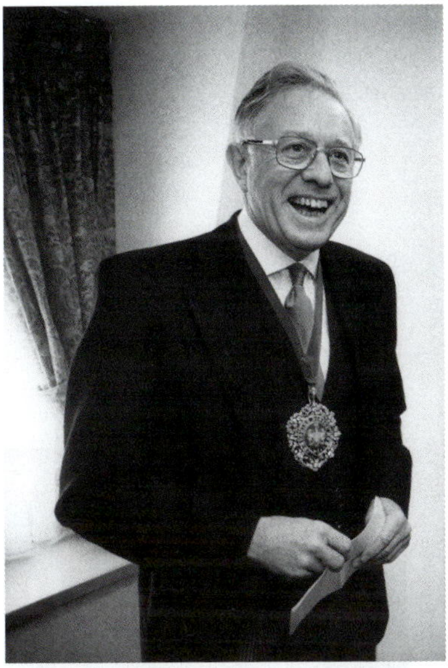

Appendix 9: Celebrity openings of departmentss **167**

Figure A9.5 *Sir John Chalstrey, endoscopy unit, 26 September 1996.*

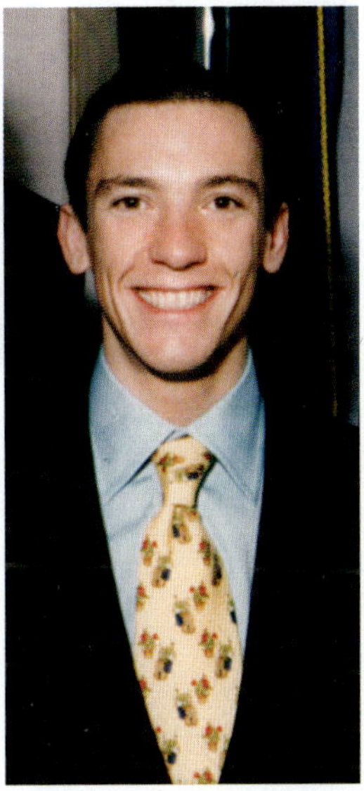

Figure A9.6 *Frankie Dettori, health screening unit, 18 November 1997.*

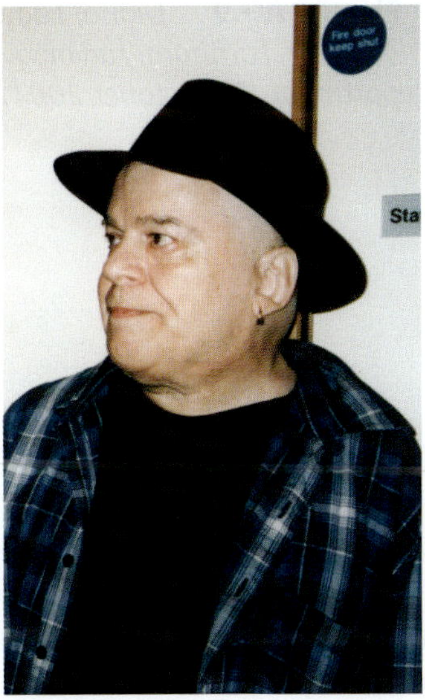

Figure A9.7 *Ian Drury, Cancerbackup, Summer 1999.*

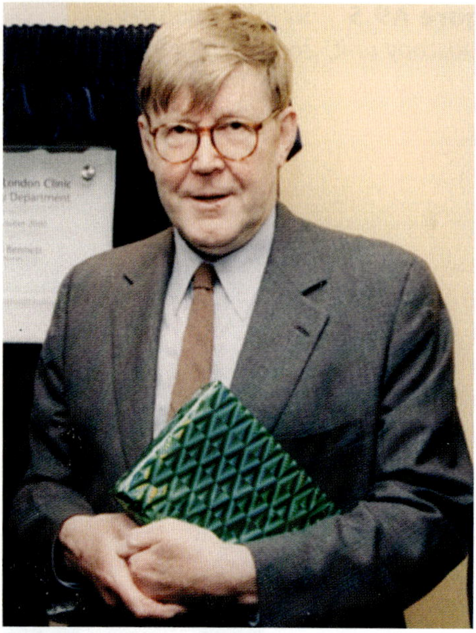

Figure A9.8 *Alan Bennett, opening of the pathology refurbishment, October 2000.*

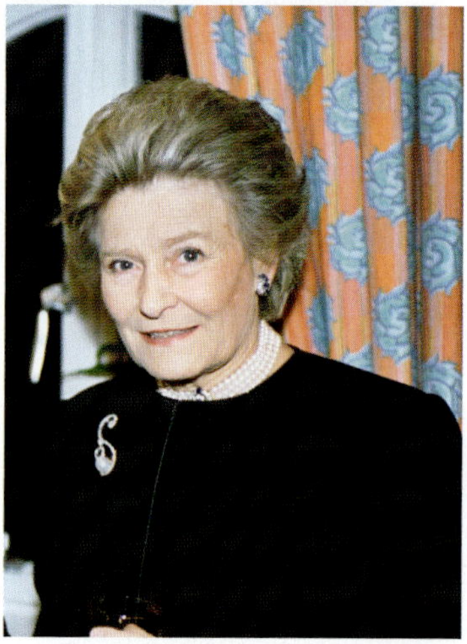

Figure A9.9 *Diana, Lady Farnham, radiology department, 25 October 2001.*

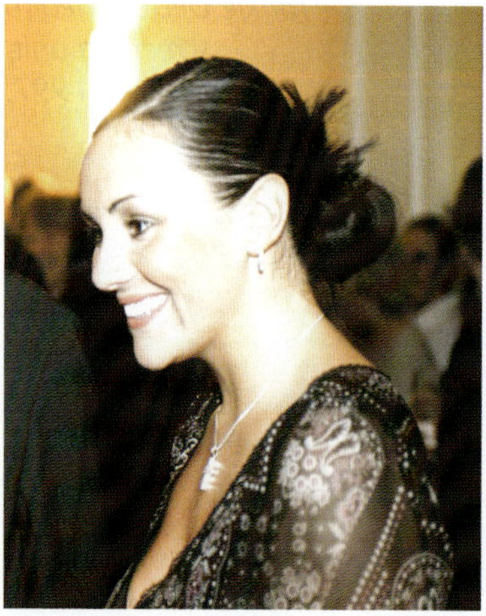

Figure A9.10 *Martine McCutcheon, 119 Harley Street, May 2002.*

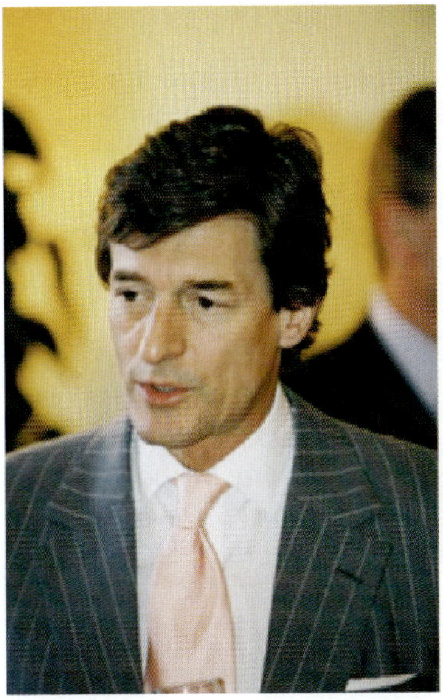

Appendix 9: Celebrity openings of departmentss **169**

Figure A9.11 *Nigel Havers, 145 Harley Street, 13 May 2003.*

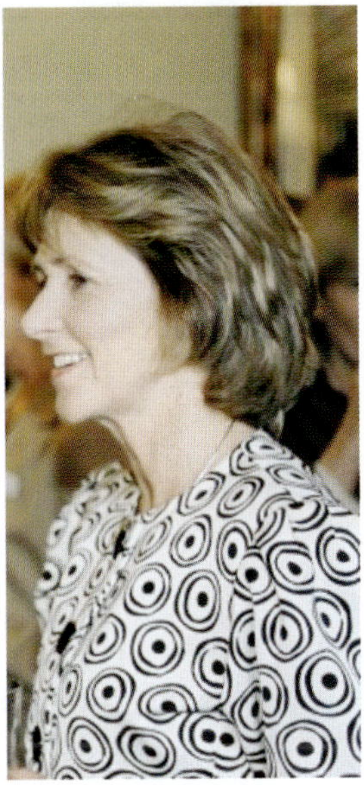

Figure A9.12 *Lady Hartington, now Duchess of Devonshire, Vernon House, September 2004.*

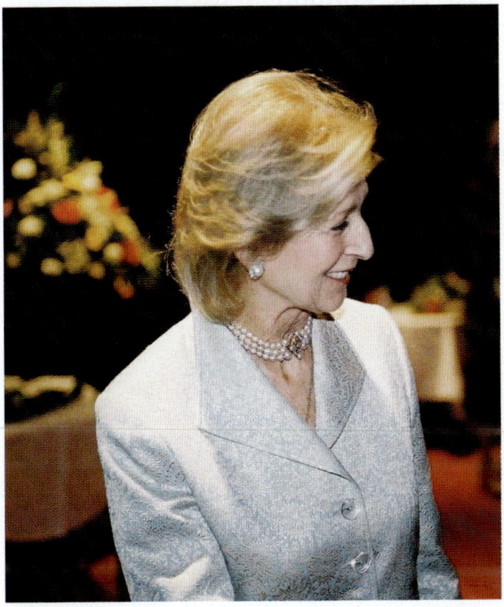

Figure A9.13 *HRH Princess Alexandra, Cancerbackup, September 2004.*

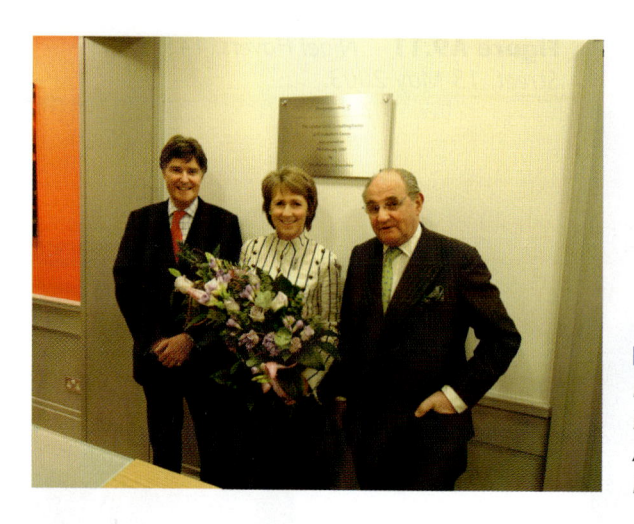

Figure A9.14 *Malcolm Miller, Duchess of Devonshire, Michael Abrahams, 5 Devonshire, Place, February 2007.*

Thursday 26th April 2007

KENSINGTON PALACE

Her Royal Highness, Patron, Prostate Research Campaign UK, this afternoon visited The London Clinic, 149 Harley Street, London W1, to view the da Vinci robot.

Box A9.1 *HRH Duchess of Gloucester, Prostate Research Campaign – da Vinci Robot, 26 April 2007. Reproduced with kind permission from the Court Circular, British Monarchy Media Centre.*

10

The London Clinic Medical Journal listings of clinical articles

Year	Volume	Issue	Title of article	Authors
1960	1	1	Viral conjunctivitis	Sir Stewart Duke-Elder GCVO, FRS
			Scope of plastic surgery	Sir Archibald McIndoe CBE, MS, FRCS, FACS
			Traumatic progressive encephalopathy of boxers	Macdonald Critchley MD, FRCP, FACP
			Smoking and the alimentary tract	F Avery Jones MD, FRCP
			The therapeutic conquest of malaria	Sir Philip Manson-Bahr CMG, DSO, MD, FRCP
			Clinical Methods: The Coboltron II (radiotherapy)	
1961	2	1	*Editorial Comment*	
			Insuring against major illness	
			Averting lazy eye	
			Prolonged chemotherapy in chronic bronchitis	
			Radio pills	
			Hearing and deafness	Terence Cawthorne FRCS
			Hypotensive anaesthesia in plastic surgery	GE Hale Enderby MB, BChir, FFARCS
			Carcinoma of the large intestine	EG Muir FRCS, MS
			Acute cerebrovascular accidents	Wylie McKissock OBE, MS, FRCS
			Varicose veins	R Rowden Foote MRCS, LRCP, DRCOG
			Clinical Methods: The freezing microtome	

Year	Volume	Issue	Title of article	Authors
1961	2	2	Editorial Comment	
			Cave Canem	
			Fallout in milk	
			Juvenile obesity	
			Precautions and errors in biliary tract surgery	Rodney Maingot FRCS
			Cancer of the pancreas	Rodney Smith MS, FRCS
			General practitioners and private beds	John H Hunt MD, MRCP
			The choice of antibiotic	D Geraint James MD, MRCP
1962	3	1	Editorial Comment	
			Fibrinolysin against cancer	
			Experience with PBI	
			Born without limbs (thalidomide deformities)	
			Diagnosing Toxoplasmosis	
			Serum protein-bound iodine (PBI) and thyroid function	HFW Kirkpatrick PhD, ARCS, DIC, FRIC
			The modern management of diabetes	Wilfrid Oakley MD, FRCP
			Acute respiratory failure	R Atwood Beaver FFA, DA
			Radioactive isotopes in medicine	Robert J Dickson MD, DMRT (Eng)
			A short history of intracranial aneurysms	James Bull MD, FRCP, FFR
1963	4	1	Editorial Comment	
			Cortisone – with care	
			Early detection of cervical cancer	
			Towards safer vaccination	
			RD Lawrence	
			Investigation and treatment of thyroid disorders	Robert J Dickson, MD, DMRT (Eng)
			Frozen shoulder	Ronald Furlong FRCS
			Pilonidal sinus	James O Robinson MD, MChir, FRCS
			Some observations on anaemia of pregnancy	Gordon Bourne FRCS, MRCOG
			Corneal grafting methods and indications	Stephen Miller MD, FRCS

Appendix 10: LCMJ listings of clinical articles

1963, Vol 4, No 2

- *Editorial Comment*
- Hormonal influence in glaucoma — Harland Rees MCh, FRCS
- Surgery for the 'liverish' — F Avery Jones MD, FRCP
- Difficulties in diagnosing cardiac pain
- Some aspects of female urology
- Gastroscopy
- Case records
- Isotopes in haematological and related studies — Richard Hunter MD, MRCP, DPM
- Leprosy and its management in Britain — Robert J Dickson MD, DMRT (Eng)
- Clinical Methods: Actinic coagulation — WH Jopling FRCPE, MRCP, DTMH

1964, Vol 5, No 1

- *Editorial Comment*
- Respiratory Failure
- Folic Acid for Abruptio Placentae?
- Disorders of the small bowel
- Antidepressants – with care
- Burns and their treatment — Robin Beare FRCS
- Parkinsonism: aetiology and treatment — JW Aldren Turner DM, FRCP
- Arteriography — Norman L Mills DMRD, MRCS, LRCP
- The indurated leg — R Rowden Foote FICS, MRCS, LRCP, DRCOG
- Therapeutic uses of radioactive isotopes — Robert J Dickson MD, DMRT (Eng)

1964, Vol 5, No 2

- *Editorial Comment*
- Congenital defects and 5-T
- Poisonous pets
- The resurgent trachoma virus
- Surgery in chronic middle ear disease
- Ageing of the skin — Stephen Gold MD, FRCP
- The delayed reader and the paediatrician — Alfred White Franklin FRCP
- Subarachnoid haemorrhage — Alan Richardson FRCS
- Congenital dislocation of the hip — TG Barlow BSc, FRCS

Year	Volume	Issue	Title of article	Authors
1965	6	1	Editorial Comment	
			Human growth hormone	JD Fergusson MD, FRCS
			The 'subclavian steal' syndrome	JR Armstrong MD, MCh, FRCS
			Cardiac resuscitation	W Ogilvie Macfeat MB, ChB, DMR
			Peritoneal dialysis	Ian P Todd MS, MD, FRCS
			Conservative treatment of prostatic cancer	Basil Kiernander MRCP, DMRE, DPhysMed
			The pathology of lumbar disc lesions	Lilian Pollard TCSP
			Case records	
			Causes of megabowel	
			The role of physical medicine in rehabilitation	
1965	6	2	Editorial Comment	
			Intensive care of acute myocardial infarction	AW Spence MD, FRCP
			Success in treating chorionepithelioma	HE Lockhart-Mummery MD, MChir, FRCS
			Protecting the haemophiliac	Patrick Clarkson MBE, FRCS
			The urethra in childhood	Robert IW Ballantine MRCS, LRCP, DA, FFA, RCS
			Hirsutism	Lawson McDonald MD, FRCP
			Polyps of the large bowel	
			Appearance, cosmetic surgery and mental health	
			Clinical Methods: The anaesthetist's first visit	
			Management of cardiac arrhythmias	
1966	7	1	Editorial Comment	
			Transferable antibiotic resistance	Charles Drew MVO, VRD, FRCS
			The irritable bowel syndrome	RMB MacKenna MD, FRCP
			Exposure to asbestos and malignancy	GD Hadley MD, FRCP
			Bypassing the blocked tube	
			Profound hypothermia in cardiac surgery	
			Rosacea	
			Clinical Methods: Gastrophotography	

Appendix 10: LCMJ listings of clinical articles

Year	Issue	Article	Author(s)
1966	7	The artificial kidney	AR Harrison MD, MRCP
		Urinary diversion in carcinoma of the bladder	Howard G Hanley MD, FRCS
		Complications and sequelae of thyroid surgery	RS Murley MS, FRCS
	2	*Editorial Comment*	
		Biochemical research in schizophrenia	
		Host-finding by mosquitos	
		Gastrin	
		Problems of maternal rubella	
		Pre-glaucoma and its diagnosis	Stephen JH Miller MD, FRCS
		Diaphragmatic hernia	Norman Tanner MD, FRCS
		Clothing dermatitis	Harold Wilson MD, FRCP
		Clinical Methods: Radiology of the urinary system	RSC Couch MD, MRCP, FFR
		Wound healing and fistula-in-ano	Henry R Thompson FRCS
		Circulating cancer cells in surgery	John D Griffiths MS, FRCS
1967	8	*Editorial Comment*	
		Treatment with iron preparations	
		Congenital night blindness	
		Intestinal cell carcinoma of the stomach	
		Renal papillary necrosis and analgesic abuse	
		Scintiscanning of the liver and pancreas	
	1	The management of chronic bronchitis	Neville C Oswald TD, MD, FRCP
		Clinical methods: Operative cholangiography	James O Robinson MD, MChir, FRCS
		Surgery of the ischaemic lower limb	FB Cockett MS FRCS
		Lumbar spinal fusion	Walter Robinson FRCS Edin
		Surgery of atrial septal defect	IM Hill MS, FRCS
1967	9	*Editorial Comment*	
		The prevention of Rh haemolytic disease	
		Erythropoietin	
	2	*Jejunal diverticulosis and B12 deficiency*	
		Are isometric exercises safe?	

Year	Volume	Issue	Title of article	Authors
1967	2	(contd.)	Vertigo and the ear	Sir Terence Cawthorne MD, FRCS
			Diversion of the portal blood	Alan H Hunt DM, MCh, FRCS
			Some aspects of bladder function in health and disease	KED Shuttleworth MS, FRCS
			Regional renal hypothermia	JEA Wickham MS, BSc, FRCS
1968	9	1	*Editorial Comment*	
			Practical care of the acute coronary patient	
			Radio-immunoassay in endocrinology	
			Surgery in mitral valve disease	Sir Thomas Holmes Sellors DM, MCH, FRCS, FRCP
			Deafness after head injuries	John Ballantyne FRCS
			Simple obesity in adults	AW Spence MD, FRCP
			Management of leukaemia	TAJ Prankerd MD, FRCP
			Corticosteroid therapy (1): clinical applications	CWH Havard DM, MRCP
1968	9	2	*Editorial Comment:*	
			Transplantation in mice and men	
			A novel anticoagulant from viper venom	
			Carbenoxolone	
			Dietary indiscretion and migraine	
			The investigation of the solitary fit	Denis Williams CBE, MD, DSc, FRCP
			Clinical Methods: Cryotherapy in ophthalmology	Stephen JH Miller MD, FRCS
			Lymphangiography	Louis Kreel MD, MRCP, FFR
			Transrectal fine-needle biopsy in diagnosing prostatic cancer	JP Williams MChir FRCS
			Corticosteroid therapy (2): complications	CWH Havard DM, MRCP
1969	10	1	*Editorial Comment*	
			Lipids and coronary prevention	
			Steroids and glaucoma	
			Measuring the cerebral blood flow	
			Lumbar puncture reviewed	

Year	Vol	Issue	Article	Author
1969	10		Management of postcricoid and cervical oesophageal cancer	DFN Harrison MD, MS, FRCS
			Selective angiography	Brian Kendall MRCP, FFR
			Congenital stenosis and atresia of the jejunum and ileum	JD Atwell FRCS
			The history of otosclerosis surgery	Sir Terence Cawthorne MD, FRCS
				Harold Ludman FRCS
		2	*Editorial Comment*	
			The future of interferon	
			Deep vein thrombosis	
			Prostaglandins	
			Management of postoperative pancreatic complications	Rodney Maingot FRCS
			Surgery of ischaemic heart disease	Stuart C Lennox FRCS
			Clinical Methods: Cardiac arrest	Alan Gilston MB, FFARCS
			The management of stroke	John Marshall MD, FRCPE, FRCP, DPM
			Management of diabetic retinopathy	Patrick Holmes Sellors FRCS
1970	11	1	*Editorial Comment*	
			L-dopa and parkinsonism	
			Asthma and hypnotherapy	
			Waiting for Fidler et al.	
			A commentary on peptic ulcer	F Avery Jones MD, FRCP
			Results of aortic or mitral valve replacement by prosthesis	John Hamer MD, PhD, FRCP
			Clinical Methods: Clinical thermography	KD Patil MB, FRCS, FRCSEd
			Salivary gland surgery: some personal reflections	David H Patey MS, FRCS
			Origins of proptosis	Harvey Jackson FRCS
1970	11	2	*Editorial Comment*	
			Anaemia and health	
			Serum hepatitis as a professional risk	
			The future of antiviral chemotherapy	

Year	Volume	Issue	Title of article	Authors
1970	12	1 *(contd.)*	Peripheral pain in the arm	Ronald Furlong FRCS
			The surgery of peptic ulcer	James O Robinson MD, MChir, FRCS
			Clinical Methods: Mammography	Norman L Mills DMRD, MRCS, LRCP
			Speech disorders in children	F Clifford Rose MRCP, DCH
			Hypospadias	JP Reidy FRCS, MD
1971	12	1	*Editorial Comment*	
			Fresh approaches to transplantation	
			Results of treating hypertension	
			The use of prostaglandins in obstetrics	
			When the migraine patient seeks help	JN Blau MD, FRCP
			The comparative pathology of tumours in man and domestic animals	Arnold Levene MB, PhD, FRCS
			Replacement of the hip joint	Peter R French FRCS
			Back-door doctor: a study in private enterprise	Col ES Phipson CIE, DSO, MD, FRCP

11

The London Clinic Medical Journal listings of non-clinical articles

Year	Volume	Issue	Title of article
1960	1	1	Introduction to first issue by Lord Evans and Sir Aynsley Bridgland, mention of Rodney Maingot as Chairman of Editorial Committee Obituary: Sir Archibald Hector McIndoe
1961	2	1	Obituary: Sir Harold Delf Gillies Obituary: Conrad Meredyth Hinds Howell
1963	4	2	Editorial comment on Sir Aynsley Bridgland with Certificate of Esteem
1964	5	1	Obituary: Lord Evans
1965	6	1	Obituary: Sir Henry Souttar
1966	7	2	Obituary: Sir Aynsley Bridgland
		2	Obituary: Dr Ronald Couch
1967	8	1	Obituary: Sir Philip Manson-Bahr
1968	9	2	Concentration of Hands (Dame Barbara Hepworth)
1969	10	1	Obituary: Mr Vincent Alpe Grantham, Chairman of Board of Governors Hands Operating (Dame Barbara Hepworth) The Scalpel (Dame Barbara Hepworth)
	10	2	As Others See Us (Dame Barbara Hepworth)
1970	11	1	Clinic News Edward Grainger Muir created knight bachelor
		2	Obituary: Sir Terence Cawthorne
1971	12	1	Obituary: Lady Bridgland

12

Obituary of Sir Aynsley Bridgland

OBITUARY

SIR AYNSLEY BRIDGLAND, C.B.E.
1893-1966

Sir Aynsley Bridgland, chairman of the Governors of London Clinic, and a dynamic force in several important companies in the City of London and elsewhere, died on 20 July, 1966, a patient in the medical centre that he had served so valuably for 31 years. He was 73.

Aynsley Vernon Bridgland was born on 24 May, 1893, the son of a businessman connected with the building industry in Adelaide, Australia. Educated at University High School, Melbourne, and the University of Adelaide, he became in the first instance a civil engineer. As such he did pioneering work while a young man in the outback, under conditions of great physical hardship. During the First World War he served as an officer in the Machine Gun Corps with the Australian forces on the Western Front.

A flair for mathematics, which was there from the outset, led him to enter the world of finance, and for some years he acted as a representative in Australia of the American oil magnate and philanthropist, John D. Rockefeller. In 1929 Bridgland decided to try his fortune in Britain.

At that stage his special interest lay in housing projects, particularly large blocks of flats, one of his earliest associates being Sir Cyril Black, M.P., now head of the Temperance Permanent Building Society and many property companies. As founder and chairman of Haleybridge Investment Trust, Ltd. and of Regis Property Co., Ltd. he left his mark on the London scene. Among the large office blocks for whose erection he was responsible are Plantation House, Bucklersbury House, Temple Court and the new International Headquarters of the Salvation Army in the City of London, not to mention Exchange Buildings in Liverpool, Regis House in Cape Town, and the first block that marked the development of Knightsbridge, London, as a business office district. In these enterprises he was closely associated with the late Lord Kennet and Mr V. A. Grantham, chairman of the Chartered Bank.

A historic discovery came to light in 1954 when the foundations of Bucklersbury House in Queen Victoria Street were being excavated; ruins uncovered by the workmen were pronounced by Professor W. F. Grimes, then Keeper of the London Museum, to be one of the temples dedicated to the ancient Persian sun god Mithras whose mystical rites were especially favoured by the Roman legions from the first century B.C. onwards.

As announcements of further discoveries of buried treasures were made by the national Press there was an enormous demand for facilities to visit

THE LONDON CLINIC MEDICAL JOURNAL

the excavation site. According to an account by Mr Ralph Merrifield, some 35,000 people were admitted during the week it was made open to the public, and many more were turned away after it had finally to be closed. Questions were asked in the House of Commons, the site was formally inspected by the Minister of Works, and a public demand arose for the preservation of the temple. Mr Bridgland's solution was to have the building company involved—Legenland Property—put up most of the money to have the remains of the temple removed and reconstructed on a neighbouring site. Winston Churchill thanked him by letter for his part in preserving and reconstructing the Mithraic Temple.

Sir Aynsley was founder and president of the Golf Society of Great Britain and arranged for it to have a first class base at Prince's Golf Links, Sandwich, a derelict waste during the war, which he was responsible for having re-created as a championship course. A keen golfer all his life, he was at one time a 'scratch' player, and won the Jubilee Vase at St Andrew's in 1959. Most of the great golfers of his day were known to him; so intrigued was he by the different methods of play and instruction that he set up a team of anatomists, physiologists, physicists, ballistics experts and other specialists to investigate the golf swing scientifically. That work is still in progress.

To most readers of this journal founded by him in 1960—and in the press at the time of his death—Sir Aynsley was best known as the man who made a success of the London Clinic. His association began in 1935, three years after it had been built by a public company under the chairmanship of the Duke of Atholl and supported by a group of 37 doctors. The enterprise ran into serious difficulties owing to under-capitalization, then A. V. Bridgland came forward with a plan. His solution was to set up and finance a company on somewhat the same lines as the Wellcome Trust to conduct the Clinic as a non-profit charity—and such it has remained. His co-trustees were Mr E. R. D. Hoare, later succeeded by Sir Tom Hickinbotham, and Mr V. A. Grantham whose wise counsel as a Governor has continued unremittingly ever since.

A. V. Bridgland did not build the London Clinic, but it will surely have pride of place among the monuments by which he will be remembered. His self-appointed task of rescuing the Clinic and promoting its interests was not merely the hobby of a wealthy man; he made of it a dedication. To that task he applied all the acumen and far-sightedness that had brought him success in commerce. It must have been a considerable satisfaction indeed to himself and his co-trustees that over the long years they succeeded in creating the premier private hospital in the British Commonwealth.

THE LONDON CLINIC MEDICAL JOURNAL

During that time the doctors who made use of the Clinic lacked nothing in the way of up-to-date equipment, for as soon as any promising new diagnostic or therapeutic technique had proved its worth the Chairman was anxious that 'his' patients should get the benefit of the advance. The 'Bridgie' that presided at 20 Devonshire Place may have had no medical training but he was *almost* a doctor. Perhaps he changed personalities as he went, but at least while he was working at the Clinic he seemed to think like a doctor—and even at times talk like one. A consultant attending him during his last illness was touched to find that in addition to a bedside Bible his reading matter on Friday mornings included *The Lancet* and *British Medical Journal*.

Sir Aynsley Bridgland presented a bluff and breezy façade that might have misled the imperceptive. In fact, he was an extremely kind man, though he would not thank you for saying so. Nor did he wish to have his many benefactions noised abroad.

Among friends who contributed to this note, one of his closest business associates suggests as an epitaph the lines of Adam Lindsay Gordon (1833-1870) which run:

> *Question not, but live and labour*
> *Till yon goal be won,*
> *Helping every feeble neighbour*
> *Seeking help from none;*
> *Life is mostly froth and bubble,*
> *Two things stand like stone,*
> *Kindness in another's trouble,*
> *Courage in your own.*

Sir Aynsley was a good man, whose passing will be mourned by many. Our profound sympathy goes out to his family who have suffered a cruel loss. With his death the London Clinic has lost its best friend; the world in which he moved will be a poorer place without him.

Reproduced with kind permission from The London Clinic Medical Journal *1966;* **7**: *15–18.*

13

Explosive ordnance threat assessment of the London Clinic Cancer Centre

(Reproduced on following pages)

THE LONDON CLINIC THE LONDON CLINIC CANCER CENTRE

This document is of UK origin and is © BACTEC International Limited. It contains proprietary information which is disclosed for the purposes of assessment and evaluation only. The contents of this document shall not in whole or in part: (i) be used for any other purpose, (ii) be disclosed to any member of the recipient's organisation not having a need to know such information nor to any third party individual, organisation or government, (iii) be stored in any retrieval system nor be reproduced or transmitted in any form by photocopying or any optical, electronic, mechanical or other means, without the prior written permission of the Managing Director, BACTEC International Limited, 37 Riverside, Sir Thomas Longley Road, Rochester, Kent ME2 4DP, United Kingdom.

EXPLOSIVE ORDNANCE THREAT ASSESSMENT

OF

THE LONDON CLINIC CANCER CENTRE

FOR

THE LONDON CLINIC

8936TA   6th JANUARY 2006

Appendix 13: Explosive ordance threat assessment etc. **187**

THE LONDON CLINIC *THE LONDON CLINIC CANCER CENTRE*

DISTRIBUTION

Copy Number   Recipient

1.   The London Clinic
2.   The London Clinic
3.   BACTEC International Limited

Date of Issue   6th January 2006   Copy No 1

THE LONDON CLINIC　　　　　　　　　　　　THE LONDON CLINIC CANCER CENTRE

EXECUTIVE SUMMARY

The Site: Is situated in the London Borough of Westminster and is located approximately 2.5 kilometres (km) north-west of the River Thames. Regents Park is located approximately 180 metres (m) to the north while Hyde Park is approximately 1.7km to the south-west. The site is centred on the National Grid Reference 528483E, 182091N.

Proposed Works: Are to include the demolition of four of the five properties located on the site and the construction of a new building with a basement level of approximately 15 metres (m) below ground level. A tunnel linking the new building and the existing London Clinic is also proposed.

Bombing History: During the Blitz of 1940-41 London was heavily bombed by the Luftwaffe. Bomb census maps show one bomb strike on the site with numerous others in the vicinity. Luftwaffe targets in the area included Euston and Paddington stations to the east and west of the site and a power station and rail marshalling yard to the north.

Explosive Ordnance Risk Assessment: BACTEC believes that there is a **medium to high** risk of encountering explosive ordnance in the northern portion of the site (Area A) and a **low to medium** risk in the southern portion (Area B) during the intrusive works associated with the development at the London Clinic Cancer Centre. This assessment is based on the following facts:

a. The site was situated in the London Borough of St Marylebone in Central London which was heavily bombed during WWII and which contained several important Luftwaffe targets such as Paddington and Euston Stations and a power station and rail marshalling yards.

b. The available bomb census maps for the area show one bomb strike on the site itself and numerous strikes in the surrounding vicinity.

c. The war damage map for the area, compiled post war, shows that the buildings on the site sustained no bomb damage during the war. However, if damage was repaired prior to 1945 it was not included on these maps.

d. There is a conflict between when building number 62 Marylebone High Street/13 Marylebone Road was constructed (the building is stated as being built in either the 1920's or 1950's). This is most probably due to the building being damaged by the recorded bomb strike and subsequently repaired.

e. The bomb strike recorded in the north-west corner of the site would have created an amount of rubble. It is possible that subsequent bombing raids may have delivered ordnance into this rubble and these went unnoticed at the time. Given the offset of a HE bomb can be up to 15m from its entry point, a risk remains of UXBs remaining in situ in areas that have not been subject to post war intrusive works.

f. Anti-Aircraft Artillery (AAA) batteries would have been deployed around the area to defend strategic positions. Unexploded AAA shells have been recovered from building sites in Central London since WWII. There remains the possibility, albeit slight, that AAA shells may have penetrated rubble on site unnoticed and therefore remain a threat to works today.

g. Since the end of WWII construction has occurred on site, however there are no records to indicate that the construction areas were certified free from explosive ordnance. Thus WWII-era UXO may remain on site.

h. The developmental works on the site will occur adjacent to industrial areas and densely populated areas of London. A detonation of a German HE UXB would be a significant incident. Apart from the danger to equipment and personnel conducting the works, the general public would also be at risk.

8936TA 06/01/06　　　　　　　　　　　　　　　　　　　　　　　*BACTEC International Limited*

Appendix 13: Explosive ordance threat assessment etc.

THE LONDON CLINIC   THE LONDON CLINIC CANCER CENTRE

Risk Mitigation Measures: Taking into account the findings of this study and the known extent of the proposed works BACTEC considers the following risk mitigation measures appropriate to support the future intrusive works at the London Clinic Cancer Centre.

All Intrusive Works

- *Explosive Ordnance Safety and Awareness Briefings to all personnel conducting intrusive works.*

Ground Clearance & Open Excavations

Area A:

- *Explosive Ordnance Disposal (EOD) Engineer Presence on Site to monitor all open excavations to a maximum bomb penetration depth.*

- *Intrusive Magnetometer Survey of all Pile locations down to a maximum bomb penetration depth and target investigation if required.*

Area B:

- *Explosive Ordnance Disposal (EOD) Engineer On-Call during excavations to the maximum bomb penetration depth.*

THE LONDON CLINIC *THE LONDON CLINIC CANCER CENTRE*

CONTENTS

DISTRIBUTION		ii
EXECUTIVE SUMMARY		iii
CONTENTS		v
ANNEXES		vii
1.	**INTRODUCTION**	1
1.1.	Background	1
1.2.	Legislation	2
1.3.	Aim	2
2.	**THREAT ASSESSMENT METHODOLOGY**	2
2.1.	Report Structure	2
2.2.	Sources of Information	3
2.3.	Historical Information	3
3.	**SITE**	4
3.1.	Site Location	4
3.2.	Site Description	4
4.	**SCOPE OF THE PROPOSED WORKS**	4
4.1.	Site Investigation	4
4.2.	Proposed Works	4
5.	**GROUND CONDITIONS**	5
5.1.	Historical Ground Investigation Data	5
6.	**SITE HISTORY**	5
6.1.	General	5
7.	**GENERAL BOMBING HISTORY OF LONDON**	6
7.1.	First World War	6
7.2.	Key Events in East London During the Second World War	6
8.	**BOMBING OF THE BOROUGH OF ST MARYLEBONE**	7
8.1.	General	7
8.2.	Bombing Density Map	7
8.3.	Air Raid Precaution (ARP) Records	8
8.4.	Air Raid Precaution (ARP) WWII Bomb Census Maps	8
8.5.	War Damage Map	9
8.6.	Bombing Statistics from the Second World War	9
8.7.	Summary and Deductions	10
9.	**GERMAN AIR-DELIVERED ORDNANCE**	10

Appendix 13: Explosive ordance threat assessment etc. **191**

THE LONDON CLINIC　　　　　　　　　　THE LONDON CLINIC CANCER CENTRE

9.1.	Generic Types of German Bombs	10
9.2.	German Air-Delivered Ordnance Failure Rate	11
9.3.	Abandoned Bombs	11
9.4.	Initiation of Unexploded Bombs	11
10.	**UXB GROUND PENETRATION ASSESSMENT**	**12**
10.1.	Sources	12
10.2.	UXB Sub-Surface Trajectory	13
10.3.	Assumptions for Assessment	13
10.4.	Site Specific Assessment	13
11.	**SECOND WORLD WAR BRITISH ORDNANCE**	**14**
11.1.	Defending London	14
11.2.	Anti-Aircraft Artillery Shells	14
11.3.	Unexploded AAA Shells	14
12.	**OFFICIAL EXPLOSIVE ORDNANCE DISPOSAL ARCHIVES**	**14**
12.1.	Results from Enquiries	14
13.	**EXPLOSIVE ORDNANCE RISK ASSESSMENT**	**15**
13.1.	The Threat	15
13.2.	Risk Assessment	16
14.	**PROPOSED RISK MITIGATION METHODOLOGY**	**16**
14.1.	General	16
14.2.	Advised Risk Mitigation Measures	17
15.	**CONCLUSIONS**	**18**
15.1.	Summary	18
15.2.	Recommendations	18
16.	**BIBLIOGRAPHY**	**19**

THE LONDON CLINIC

THE LONDON CLINIC CANCER CENTRE

ANNEXES

ANNEX A   Site Location Maps

ANNEX B   2003 Aerial Photograph

ANNEX C   Site Plans

ANNEX D   WWI Bomb Plot of London

ANNEX E   War Damage Map

ANNEX F   Luftwaffe Target Reconnaissance Photograph

ANNEX G   Bomb Density Map

ANNEX H   Bomb Census Maps

ANNEX I   London Bomb Damage Photographs

ANNEX J   German Air-Delivered Ordnance

ANNEX K   Press Article Relating to Detonation of UXB During Intrusive Works

ANNEX L   Risk Map

Appendix 13: Explosive ordance threat assessment etc. **193**

THE LONDON CLINIC　　　　　　　　　　　THE LONDON CLINIC CANCER CENTRE

EXPLOSIVE ORDNANCE THREAT ASSESSMENT

OF

THE LONDON CLINIC CANCER CENTRE

FOR

THE LONDON CLINIC

JANUARY 2006

1. INTRODUCTION

1.1. Background

The London Clinic has commissioned BACTEC International Limited to conduct an Explosive Ordnance Threat Assessment for the proposed intrusive works at The London Clinic Cancer Centre. Site location maps are presented in Annex A.

During the Blitz of World War Two (WWII) the German Air Force (Luftwaffe) bombed London continuously for nine months, their objectives being to cause material destruction and break Britain's morale. The Luftwaffe aimed at civilian and economic targets, the majority of which were located in London; as a result the city was extensively bombed between 1940 and 1941.

It should be noted that a series of bombing raids had also taken place in London during the First World War (WWI). Zeppelins and 'Gotha' bombers conducted a series of attacks against Britain. The quantities of bombs cannot be compared to the Blitz of WWII, but a number did fall on Westminster. Although rare, unexploded WWI bombs are still uncovered today and remain a threat to site works. Reporting during WWI was relatively poor and few records remain today, therefore although this study recognises the threat posed by WWI munitions, it cannot be quantified to the same degree as the WWII threat.

During WWII a significant proportion of aerially delivered bombs failed to function and penetrated the ground without exploding. As a result, unexploded bombs (UXB) have been regularly encountered during intrusive construction works since the end of WWII.

Due to the advances in survey methods for the detection of unexploded ordnance (UXO) and an increased awareness, the risk of inadvertently encountering an item of ordnance has been reduced significantly. However, as with all unexploded devices, the potential consequences of an explosion are extremely severe.

1.2. Legislation

The Health & Safety at Work Act and the Construction (Design & Management) Regulations of 1994 do not specifically require a search for unexploded ordnance. However, there is an obligation on those responsible for intrusive works to ensure that comprehensive threat assessment and risk mitigation measures are taken with regard to all underground hazards on site.

1.3. Aim

The aim of this report is to identify the threat posed by unexploded ordnance during the proposed works at The London Clinic Cancer Centre and to recommend risk mitigation measures, if deemed necessary, to reduce the threat from explosive ordnance during the envisaged works.

2. THREAT ASSESSMENT METHODOLOGY

2.1. Report Structure

BACTEC have employed the following methodology in preparing this Explosive Ordnance Threat Assessment:

a. The scope of the site has been considered.

b. Ground conditions were examined and summarised.

c. The scope of the proposed works has been considered.

d. The site history was considered, including previous uses.

e. The threat posed by German air-delivered ordnance has been established.

f. The effect of German air-delivered ordnance has been considered, together with the threat it poses.

Appendix 13: Explosive ordance threat assessment etc. **195**

THE LONDON CLINIC   THE LONDON CLINIC CANCER CENTRE

g. The effect of British Ordnance, and the circumstances in which it was employed to defend against enemy aircraft, has been considered together with the threat it poses.

h. The holistic Unexploded Ordnance (UXO) threat was considered, including the types that could be encountered, the probabilities of encountering them as well as exposing the potential mechanisms and risks of detonation.

i. The risks regarding explosive ordnance have been assessed.

j. Risk mitigation measures are presented.

k. Conclusions have been drawn and recommendations made.

2.2. Sources of Information

BACTEC has carried out detailed historical research for this Explosive Ordnance Threat Assessment. Military records and archived material held both in the public domain and Ministry of Defence (MoD) sources were consulted. Information was also obtained from the following sources.

a. The National Archives (formerly Public Record Office), London.

b. The Explosive Ordnance Disposal (EOD) Archive Information office at 33 Engineer Regiment (EOD).

c. The London Clinic has provided geotechnical information, historical maps, proposed construction details and a site plan.

d. BACTEC's in-house historical database.

e. BACTEC's in-house library which includes books, media articles and internet-based material.

2.3. Historical Information

It should be noted that the accuracy of wartime records and maps in terms of location, quantity and nature of ordnance cannot be verified and therefore needs to be considered as part of the overall explosive ordnance risk analysis.

During an enemy air raid it was quite possible that mistakes were made in counting the number of bombs dropped against detonations. Records were often made immediately after a raid, at which time the full extent of the raid was not determined as priority was given to casualties and damage limitation. Records of raids that took place on sparsely or uninhabited areas also tended to be inaccurate and were often based upon third party or hearsay information.

Experience has shown that, in general, records made during the war were only as accurate as time and information permitted. Some wartime reports mention that detailed records of certain air attacks (particularly those on military and industrial targets) were not maintained, or were held separately by the relevant authorities, for security and strategic reasons. For these reasons it is to be expected that historic bomb plots will be incomplete, and they cannot be independently verified. This is borne out by the number of unrecorded bombs that have been found since the war.

3. SITE

3.1. Site Location

The site is situated in the London Borough of Westminster and is located approximately 2.5 kilometres (km) north-west of the river Thames. Regents Park is located approximately 180 metres (m) to the north while Hyde Park is approximately 1.7km to the south-west. The A41 Marylebone Road bounds the site to the north with Marylebone High Street bounding the site to the east. Devonshire Place bounds the site to the west. The site is centred on the National Grid Reference 528483E, 182091N. Site location maps are presented in Annex A.

3.2. Site Description

The site comprises five structures that front onto Devonshire Place, Marylebone High Street and Marylebone Road and are of varying dates of construction. The main London Clinic building, a multi-storey block, fronts onto Marylebone Road and Devonshire Place. The five structures are of differing sizes and surround a basement level courtyard. A 2003 aerial photograph illustrating the site is presented in Annex B.

4. SCOPE OF THE PROPOSED WORKS

4.1. Site Investigation

BACTEC is unaware of any proposed site investigation to be undertaken within the site boundary

4.2. Proposed Works

The proposed works are to include the demolition of four of the five structures that front onto Marylebone High Street, Devonshire Place and Marylebone Road. Number 23 Devonshire Place is a listed Georgian building and is to be retained and refurbished internally. The demolition is to be carried out to basement slab level, approximately 2.5 metres below ground level (m bgl). A new building is to be constructed on the site incorporating number 23 Devonshire Place. To construct the basement for the new build a series of piles will be sunk around the perimeter of the site, with the enclosed area being excavated to 15m bgl. As the excavation progresses temporary propping will hold the piles in place. When the excavation phase is complete the main foundation piles will be sunk, after which the new building will be constructed back out of the hole with the floor propping the piles to the perimeter. A tunnel, connecting the London Clinic with the new build at basement level, is then to be constructed beneath Devonshire Place. Site plans

Appendix 13: Explosive ordance threat assessment etc. **197**

THE LONDON CLINIC   THE LONDON CLINIC CANCER CENTRE

showing the buildings to be demolished and the new build perimeter and proposed tunnel location are presented in Annex C.

5. GROUND CONDITIONS

5.1. Historical Ground Investigation Data

Ground investigation comprising 6 boreholes and 12 trial pits was undertaken between June and October 2005 by Alan Baxter and Associates. The geology encountered during the ground investigation is as follows:

MADE GROUND: To a maximum depth of 3.20 m bgl.

SAND: Brown slightly clayey fine to coarse with fine to medium fine gravel to 2.80 m bgl. (Encountered in borehole 1 only).

GRAVEL: Dense to medium dense brown and yellow fine to coarse gravel to a maximum depth of 6.0m bgl.

LONDON CLAY: Encountered to depths of approximately 35.0m bgl.

Boreholes did not exceed 43.0 m bgl; the Lambeth Group was encountered at depths of approximately 32m bgl.

6. SITE HISTORY

6.1. General

Historical maps showing the site in 1824 and 1913 were provided by the London Clinic. The maps are of little use for the purposes of this desk study (and are not included as an annex) but show the site was free of structures in 1824 except for number 23 Devonshire Place which is believed to have been constructed in 1793. The main London Clinic building was constructed between 1932 and 1936.

Annex C details the buildings on site to be demolished; these are thought to date from the following:

- The 'block' next to 17 Devonshire Place is an extension to the main building and was constructed in the early 1970's on piled foundations.

- 58 Marylebone High Street is a small office building constructed in the late 1960's.

- Ferguson House, across Marylebone High Street from the site, is a late 1960's early 1970's building.

- 22 Devonshire Place was constructed in the 1920's to 1930's.

8936TA 06/01/06   *BACTEC International Limited*

- 21 Devonshire Place was constructed in 1959.

- 62 Marylebone High Street/13 Marylebone Road – either built in the 1920's or possibly 1950's (**See section 8.4 below**) the same as 21 Devonshire Place next door.

- 60 Marylebone High Street was built in the 1920's.

- A single extension to the rear of 23 Devonshire Place was built in the 1900's.

All the buildings have basements to approximately 2.5m bgl.

7. GENERAL BOMBING HISTORY OF LONDON

7.1. First World War

London suffered aerial bombardment during WWI. This began with Zeppelins bombing the area indiscriminately during a series of night raids. On 13th June 1917 the first daylight aerial bombing of London by fixed-wing aircraft occurred. These Gotha bombers killed and injured more than 500 people. A WWI bomb plot is presented at Annex D. As the scale of the map is small it is difficult to determine the exact boundary of the site; however there are recorded bomb strikes to the east of Portland Place approximately 200m away. There are no recorded bomb strikes on the site itself. It should be noted that the map cannot be considered definitive in view of the poor reporting of incidents during WWI. Additional bombs may have fallen in this area but went unnoticed and/or unrecorded.

The closest documented Zeppelin raid to the site (approximately 2 km to the east) occurred on the evening of 13th October 1915 at Gray's Inn Road when several incendiaries and high explosives were dropped.

7.2. Key Events in East London During the Second World War

At the start of WWII, the Luftwaffe planned to destroy key military locations, i.e. Naval installations and Royal Air Force (RAF) airfields, during a series of daylight bombing raids. These tactics were soon modified to include both economic and industrial sites. Targets included railway infrastructure, power stations, weapon manufacturing plants and gas works. Daylight raids were reduced, in favour of attacking targets under the cover of darkness.

As the war progressed civilians in large towns and cities (most notably London) became the principle focus of the Luftwaffe and high altitude 'carpet' bombing was employed. By May 1941, the concentrated attacks on London ceased as the Luftwaffe aircraft were diverted to other towns and cities in Britain. Nevertheless sporadic bombing of London continued throughout WWII.

Throughout WWII a total of 71 'major' air raids took place on London, resulting in 29,000 people killed and 50,000 injured. An estimated 190,000 bombs (including incendiaries and anti-personnel bombs) were dropped, equivalent to 18,000 tons.

From 1943 to 1945 there was the additional hazard of unmanned rockets and missiles (known as V-Weapons) launched from aircraft bases in occupied Holland, Belgium and France as well as Germany. The most well-known of these self-propelled bombs were the V1 (Flying Bomb or Doodlebug) and the V2 (Long Range Rocket). Although the V1 and V2 caused concern to the civilian population, the body of the munition was 'thin skinned' and often broke up on impact if they failed to explode, however the 1000 kilogram (kg) warhead was contained in a 'thick skinned' body which conceivably could have penetrated the ground and gone unrecovered. However, their relatively low numbers allowed accurate records of their strikes to be maintained. The war damage map of the area (Annex E) shows five V1 Flying Bomb strikes within 800m of the site.

8. BOMBING OF THE BOROUGH OF ST MARYLEBONE

8.1. General

During WWII, the site was situated in the London Borough of St Marylebone (which later became incorporated into Westminster). Written bombing records for St Marylebone are sparse, although the bomb census maps and war damage maps for the district indicate a heavy level of bombing in the borough.

It is clear from the bomb census maps that there were numerous viable Luftwaffe targets near to the site of the proposed works. Euston Station lies approximately 1 km to the north-east and Paddington Station approximately 2km to the west. The central district of Oxford Street is approximately 1 km to the south. In addition, a designated target, seen in the Luftwaffe target reconnaissance photograph presented in Annex F, lies within 1 km of the site to the north. This target comprised a power station and rail depot with marshalling yards. The railways were recognised by the Germans' for importance to the Allied war effort and regular bombing raids were conducted to disrupt and destroy this infrastructure. There are various other large buildings and landmarks in the vicinity such as the British Museum to the south-west and the large Post Office building to the east.

Throughout WWII records of bombing incidents in London were kept by the Air Raid Precaution (ARP); Civil Defence Office and the London Port Authority. This was done not only to identify the areas affected, but also in an attempt to find patterns in the Germans' bombing strategy and thus predict where future raids may take place. These records were kept in the form of typed or hand written notes and/or presented on bomb census maps.

8.2. Bombing Density Map

The bombing density map, presented at Annex G, depicts the density of bombs that fell on Greater London throughout WWII. The highest densities were recorded around Central and East London along the River Thames.

The site is close to Central London and therefore lies in an area where bombing density was high, i.e. around 65-128 bombs dropped per square kilometre.

8.3. Air Raid Precaution (ARP) Records

Bombing records for the site have been obtained from the National Archives, and various books and internet based resources were consulted. The findings for bomb related incidents on and around the site between 1939 and 1945 are presented below:

18th February 1940 – St Marylebone district bombed with a mixture of High Explosive (HE) and Incendiary bombs.

10th September 1940 – St Marylebone bombed, large fires were reported throughout the district.

15th September 1940 – St Marylebone district bombed, the BBC was thought to be the primary target.

2nd October 1940 – St Marylebone bombed, HE bombs reported on the London and North Eastern Railway (LNER) rail line damaging 30 feet of track.

15th October 1940 – St Marylebone heavily bombed in a raid that centred around Cumberland Place (Seymour Street) which killed and injured 100 people.

8th December 1940 – St Marylebone district heavily bombed. St Marylebone Station and Tottenham Court Road heavily hit by HE bombs.

8th March 1941 – Between 2030 hours and 2300 hours 14 incidents recorded in St Marylebone centred on Coventry Street. 9 incidents due to Incendiary bombs with a further 5 due to HE bombs. 406 fires were reported of which 2 were serious requiring between 11 and 30 fire pumps, 48 were medium requiring 2-10 pumps, 356 were small requiring 1 pump. All fires were successfully extinguished. During this raid the Central London region, of which St Marylebone was a part, suffered 17 people killed with a further 13 injured.

The above ARP records were obtained from the National Archives. The number of records for this region is unusually sparse given the high level of bombing that the area sustained. It was not uncommon for records to be destroyed post-war, or even during bombing raids themselves.

8.4. Air Raid Precaution (ARP) WWII Bomb Census Maps

The bomb census maps shown at Annex H show all of the bombs recorded as landing in the vicinity of The London Clinic site during WWII. It should be noted that bomb census maps do not distinguish between the type or size of bombs or whether or not they exploded. The maps highlight the intensity of bombing that occurred in the area of the site, with numerous bomb strikes shown.

One bomb is recorded as falling on the site in the north-western corner between 5/5/1941 and 12/5/1941. This bomb is plotted as falling on number 62 Marylebone High Street/13 Marylebone Road and may be responsible for the destruction of this building. This may explain why there is some discrepancy between the known dates

Appendix 13: Explosive ordance threat assessment etc. **201**

THE LONDON CLINIC   THE LONDON CLINIC CANCER CENTRE

of this building's construction (**as detailed in section 6.1 above**). Damage caused by this bomb strike may have required total or partial reconstruction of the building; in other words it is probably of a 1920's date with post-war reconstruction.

Bombs also fell on Harley Street and Devonshire Mews West, to the south and south-west of the site, Park Crescent and Devonshire Street, to the east and York Terrace to the north. The bomb damage photographs presented in Annex I illustrate how items of ordnance could penetrate bomb damage rubble unnoticed during a raid.

8.5. War Damage Map

The war damage map shows the level of damage caused to buildings by ordnance during WWII; it also depicts the locations of V1 and V2 rocket strikes.

- **War Damage Map:** The London war damage map for this area (number 49), which was compiled after the war, is presented in Annex E. It is apparent that there was a significant concentration of bomb damage to the east, west and north of the site. The site itself shows no evidence of any bomb damage. Bomb damage that was incurred early in the war and was subsequently repaired prior to 1945 does not show on these maps. This may explain why the site is shown clear of damage, even though it sustained a bomb strike.

8.6. Bombing Statistics from the Second World War

The tables below summarise the German ordnance reported as falling in the London Borough of St Marylebone throughout WWII (excluding incendiary and anti-personnel bombs).

Record of German Ordnance Dropped in The London Borough of St Marylebone	
Area Acreage	1473
High Explosive Bombs (All Types)	398
Parachute Mines	6
Oil Bomb	12
Phosphorous Bomb	16
Pilotless Aircraft (V1)	0
Fire Pot	13
Long Range Rocket (V2)	2
Total	**444**
Number of items per 1000 acres	303.5

Detailed records of the quantity and locations of incendiary and anti-personnel bombs were not maintained, as they were too numerous to record. Although these are not particularly significant in the threat they pose, they nevertheless are items of ordnance that were designed to cause damage and inflict injury. This is not overlooked in assessing the general risk to personnel and equipment. Furthermore, the table above does not reflect the unexploded ordnance (UXO) found during or after WWII. The accuracy of this table cannot be verified as the information has been obtained from a single source.

8.7. Summary and Deductions

Although ARP records for the area were not comprehensive, the borough of St Marylebone did suffer heavy bombing raids in the early years of WWII. The site itself sustained a bomb strike in the north-west corner and it is suggested that this caused the reconstruction of No. 62 Marylebone High Street/13 Marylebone Road. The areas surrounding the site to the east, west, north and south all sustained bomb strikes with the closest being recorded on Park Crescent, Portland Place and on Harley Street. These are all within 200 metres (m) of the site. One bomb strike on Devonshire Mews West, to the immediate south of site, is within 50m.

The area in general held strategic targets of importance, (such as the main line stations and rail marshalling yards), for the Luftwaffe and these were repeatedly bombed in the hope of disrupting the rail system. In addition a power station to the north-west, which was photographed by reconnaissance aircraft before the war, was targeted. There are no recorded bomb strikes or bomb damage on the London Clinic main building.

9. GERMAN AIR-DELIVERED ORDNANCE

9.1. Generic Types of German Bombs

The nature and characteristics of the ordnance used by the Luftwaffe allows an informed assessment of the hazards posed by any unexploded items that may remain today. Detailed illustrations of German air delivered ordnance are presented at Annex J.

a. *HE Bombs:* In terms of weight of ordnance dropped, HE bombs are the most likely type to be encountered. Additionally, they have the weight, velocity and shape to easily penetrate the ground if they failed to explode. The post-raid surveys carried out by the fire, police and civil defence personnel may have failed to spot an entry hole or other indications that a bomb penetrated the ground and failed to explode. Where evidence was reported, the Bomb Disposal team (BD, now known as Explosive Ordnance Disposal or EOD) would have been requested to investigate.

b. *Blast Bombs/ Parachute Mines:* Blast bombs generally had a slow rate of descent and were extremely unlikely to have penetrated the ground. Non-retarded mines would have shattered on most ground types, if they had failed to explode. There have been extreme cases when these items have been found unexploded, but this was where the ground was either very soft or where standing water had reduced the impact. BACTEC does not consider there to be a significant threat from this type of munition on this site.

c. *Incendiary Bombs (IB):* IB were unlikely to penetrate the ground and would have been located on the post-raid survey. Generally IB do not contain high explosives and hence intrusive works are unlikely to cause a detonation.

d. *Anti-personnel (AP) Bomblets:* AP bombs had little ground penetration ability and should have been located by the post-raid survey.

e. *Specialist Bombs:* These types are more likely to behave as HE bombs, but do not contain high explosive and therefore a detonation consequence is unlikely.

9.2. German Air-Delivered Ordnance Failure Rate

It should be noted that generally around 10% of the German HE bombs dropped during WWII failed to explode as designed. Home Office statistics relating to unexploded ordnance for the Borough of St Marylebone were consulted. These documents indicate that the recorded failure rate for HE bombs in this Borough was lower at 7.3%.

9.3. Abandoned Bombs

A post-air raid survey of buildings, facilities and installations would have included a search for evidence of bomb entry holes. If evidence were encountered, Bomb Disposal teams would normally have been requested to attempt to locate, render safe and dispose of the bomb. Occasionally evidence of UXBs was discovered but due to a relatively benign position, access problems or as a result of a shortage of resources the UXB could not be exposed and rendered safe. Such an incident may have been recorded and noted as an *Abandoned Bomb*. There are no recorded abandoned bombs on the site.

Given the inaccuracy of WWII records and the fact that these bombs were 'abandoned', their locations cannot be considered definitive, nor exhaustive. The MoD states that 'action to make the devices safe would be taken only if it was thought they were unstable' or their location was to be developed in the future. It should be noted that other than the 'officially' abandoned bombs, there will inevitably be UXBs that were never recorded.

9.4. Initiation of Unexploded Bombs

Unexploded bombs do not spontaneously explode. All high explosive requires significant energy to create the conditions for detonation to occur. In the case of unexploded German bombs discovered within the construction site environment, there are a number of potential initiation mechanisms:

a. *Direct impact onto the main body of the bomb:* Unless the fuze or fuze pocket is struck, there needs to be a significant impact (e.g. from piling or large and violent mechanical excavation) to initiate a buried iron bomb. Such violent action can cause the bomb to detonate e.g. pile driving initiated the detonation of a WWII era bomb in Berlin in 1994 with resulting loss of life (see press report at Annex K).

b. *Re-starting the clock timer in the fuze:* Only a small proportion of German WWII bombs employed clockwork fuzes. It is probable that significant corrosion has taken place within the fuze mechanism over the last 60 years that would prevent clockwork mechanisms from functioning.

c. *Induction of a static charge, causing a current in an electric fuze:* The majority of German WWII bombs employed electric fuzes. It is probable that significant corrosion has taken place within the fuze mechanism over the last 60 years that would earth or "short" any fuze circuit.

d. *Friction impact initiating the (more sensitive) fuze explosive:* This is the most likely scenario resulting in the bomb detonating.

10. UXB GROUND PENETRATION ASSESSMENT

10.1. Sources

The study of UXB penetration into natural ground has been extensively conducted by numerous organisations since the end of WWII. The United States Army Corps of Engineers lead this research, and have conducted more than 1000 'real' bomb penetration experiments in known geology.

BACTEC International Limited has reviewed many of the most credible penetration equations and theories, and concluded that relying on a mathematical approach alone cannot guarantee an accurate bomb penetration figure. This is an inevitable consequence of the need to input a number of variables for mathematical modelling which requires assumptions on such aspects of a bombing raid as:

a. Ground conditions at time of impact, including different geological layers and level of the water table.

b. Aircraft speed at time of release of the bomb.

c. Impact angle.

d. Impact velocity.

e. Bomb dimensions.

f. Bomb mass.

Much of this information is not available or is too complex to be taken account of by the modelling.

BACTEC has found that the most appropriate way of determining the maximum penetration on any given site is to take the following approach.

- Stage One – Review the historical geotechnical data for the site or region.

- Stage Two – Study actual Bomb Disposal Officer reports from similar sites (case studies).

- Stage Three – Consult military manuals and documentation relating to UXB penetration.

Appendix 13: Explosive ordance threat assessment etc.

THE LONDON CLINIC   THE LONDON CLINIC CANCER CENTRE

- Stage Four – Conduct a site-specific computer-generated bomb penetration assessment.

- Stage Five – Assess all information generated from above to give maximum likely bomb penetration figure.

10.2. UXB Sub-Surface Trajectory

One of the most common WWII methods of identifying the presence of a UXB was the discovery of an entry hole. Even though a possible hole of entry of a bomb may have been detected, bombs rarely conform to a normal sub-surface trajectory. Many bombs describe a "j" curve, coming to rest at a considerable distance from the original hole of entry and often at a much shallower depth than one would ordinarily expect. Therefore UXB could potentially be located under a site, and at a shallow depth, even if it failed to land directly on it. The horizontal distance of a UXB from its Point of Entry is known as "offset" and a typical value for 500kg bombs is 15m.

10.3. Assumptions for Assessment

When conducting the assessment for Westminster Kingsway College, the following assumptions were used:

a. Geology – Made ground between 0.9m and 3.2m bgl, Gravels to a maximum depth of 6.0m bgl and London Clay to a depth of approximately 35.0m bgl.

b. Impact Velocity – 267 metres per second is used, as this would be generated by a high level release height typically used by the Luftwaffe.

c. Impact Angle – An angle of 80-90° from horizontal is used as worse case.

d. Bomb Mass – The 500kg SC (General Purpose) HE bomb is used as the "sample" bomb. This was the largest of the common bombs used against Britain. Note that the penetration depth of the less common 1000kg and 2000kg bombs would be somewhat greater and the smaller 250kg and 50kg lower.

e. Bomb Configuration – As above, the 500kg SC HE is used, but it is assumed for this study that no retarder units, or armour piecing nose units were fitted.

10.4. Site Specific Assessment

BACTEC International Limited has assessed that a 500kg SC HE bomb (the largest of the common bombs used against England) once it has passed through any made ground, is likely to have a maximum penetration depth of 5.0 metres below WWII ground level on the site.

11. SECOND WORLD WAR BRITISH ORDNANCE

11.1. Defending London

The main defence against enemy bombers attacking London were the fighter aircraft stationed at airfields such as West Malling, Hornchurch and Biggin Hill. Barrage balloons and Anti-Aircraft Artillery (AAA) batteries contributed towards the air defences of London. However at the start of the war London was under-protected from the bombers with only 92 anti-aircraft guns. This soon changed after the first year of heavy enemy bombing. London was finally heavily defended by numerous AAA batteries, which fired large calibre projectiles at enemy raiders.

11.2. Anti-Aircraft Artillery Shells

The AAA shells were high explosive projectiles, usually fitted with a time delay or barometric pressure fuze to make them explode at a height close to bomber formations. If these shells failed to explode or strike an aircraft, they would eventually fall back to earth. Unexploded AAA shells pose a similar threat to anti-personnel bombs in terms of blast and fragmentation hazards, and are at times mistakenly identified as small German aircraft-delivered bombs.

11.3. Unexploded AAA Shells

Unexploded AAA shells have been removed from London, during and after WWII. This type of ordnance is not likely to have had great penetration ability, and the majority of AAA shells are found close to ground level in made ground. The level of damage sustained on site increases the risk that an unexploded AAA shell fell unnoticed in the rubble and may subsequently have been backfilled into the cellars when the buildings were demolished.

12. OFFICIAL EXPLOSIVE ORDNANCE DISPOSAL ARCHIVES

12.1. Results from Enquiries

Information regarding the site was not available from the Explosive Ordnance Disposal (EOD) Archive Information Office at 33 Engineer Regiment (EOD) at the time this report was published. Once the data is available BACTEC will forward an addendum to the client if necessary.

It should be noted that the 33 Engineer Regiment is not the definitive source; it is possible that records existed of abandoned bombs or explosive ordnance activities in this area, but these records may have been missed during research or damaged, lost or destroyed since WWII.

Appendix 13: Explosive ordance threat assessment etc.   **207**

THE LONDON CLINIC   THE LONDON CLINIC CANCER CENTRE

13. EXPLOSIVE ORDNANCE RISK ASSESSMENT

13.1. The Threat

BACTEC has assessed the risk on site from UXB and, for the purposes of recommending risk mitigation measures, has divided the site into two separate areas. The northern portion of the site (Area A) has been assessed as having a medium to high risk while the southern portion (Area B) has a low to medium risk; these are illustrated in Annex L. This assessment is based on the following facts:

a. The site was situated in the London Borough of St Marylebone in Central London which was heavily bombed during WWII and which contained several important Luftwaffe targets such as Paddington and Euston Stations, rail marshalling yards and a power station.

b. The available bomb census maps for the area show one bomb strike on the north-western portion of the site and numerous strikes in the surrounding vicinity.

c. The war damage map for the area, compiled post war, shows that the buildings on the site sustained no bomb damage during the war. However, if damage was repaired prior to 1945 it was not included on these maps.

d. There is uncertainty as to when No. 62 Marylebone High Street/13 Marylebone Road was constructed. This is most probably due to the building being damaged by the recorded bomb strike on site and being subsequently repaired.

e. The bomb strike recorded in the north-west corner of the site would have created an amount of rubble. It is possible that subsequent bombing raids may have delivered ordnance into this rubble that went unnoticed at the time. Given the offset of a HE bomb can be up to 15m from its entry point (**see 10.2**), a risk remains of UXBs remaining in situ in areas that have not been subject to post war intrusive works.

f. Anti-Aircraft Artillery (AAA) batteries would have been deployed around the area to defend strategic positions. Unexploded AAA shells have been recovered from building sites in Central London since WWII. There remains the possibility, albeit slight, that AAA shells may have penetrated rubble on site unnoticed and therefore remain as a threat to works today.

g. Since the end of WWII construction has occurred in some areas of the site, however there are no records to indicate that the construction areas were certified free from explosive ordnance. Thus WWII-era UXO may remain on site.

h. The developmental works on the site will occur adjacent to industrial areas and densely populated areas of London. A detonation of a German HE UXB would be a significant incident. Apart from the danger to equipment and personnel conducting the works, the general public would also be at risk.

Area A has been classed as a medium to high risk, this is due to the recorded bomb strike on the north-west portion of the site and the threat from the 15m 'J' curve effect (as detailed in section **10.2.** and in point e. above). The made ground and gravel levels

8936TA 06/01/06   15   *BACTEC International Limited*

on site indicate the 'J' curve may be less than the 15m figure however; BACTEC uses this figure as the worst case scenario and therefore applies it to all sites when recommending risk mitigation measures. The absence of the immediate post war historical maps for the study site, detailing bomb damage, and the conflicting evidence from the bomb census map and the War Damage Map (which show a bomb strike on site but no damage respectively) means the site must be classified as a medium to high risk.

Conversely, Area B is at a lower risk from UXB due to the lack of evidence detailing any bomb strikes, war damage and the inability of a HE bomb to travel more than 15m through the underlying geology found on site.

13.2. Risk Assessment

The overall risk to the site from unexploded ordnance is derived by assessing both the probability of occurrence and the consequences of detonation. The levels of risk posed by unexploded ordnance at the London Clinic Cancer Centre development can be demonstrated in the tables below:

	Area A Level of Risk			
Type of Ordnance	Negligible	Low	Medium	High
German UXBs			*	
British AAA		*		

	Area B Level of Risk			
Type of Ordnance	Negligible	Low	Medium	High
German UXBs		*		
British AAA		*		

14. PROPOSED RISK MITIGATION METHODOLOGY

14.1. General

Taking into consideration the findings of this study and extent of the proposed intrusive works BACTEC considers the overall threat on site from UXB to be **low to medium** in Area B with a **medium to high** risk in Area A. BACTEC believes

Appendix 13: Explosive ordance threat assessment etc.

THE LONDON CLINICTHE LONDON CLINIC CANCER CENTRE

the following risk mitigation measures should be deployed to support any intrusive engineering works associated with the London Clinic Cancer Centre development:

14.2. Advised Risk Mitigation Measures

All Intrusive Works

- *Explosive Ordnance Safety and Awareness Briefings to all personnel conducting intrusive works:* A briefing is essential when there is a possibility of explosive ordnance contamination and is a vital part of the general safety requirement. All personnel working on the site should receive a general briefing on the identification of UXB, what actions they should take to keep people and equipment away from the hazard, and to alert site management. Posters and information of a general nature of the UXB threat should be held in the site office for reference and as a reminder. The safety awareness briefing is an essential part of the Health & Safety Plan for the site and conforms to the CDM regulations 1994. BACTEC is able to assist with these briefings.

Area A:

- *Explosive Ordnance Disposal (EOD) Engineer Presence on Site to Monitor All Open Excavations to a Maximum Bomb penetration Depth*: When on site the role of the EOD Engineer would include; monitoring works using visual recognition and instrumentation and immediate response to reports of suspicious objects or suspected items of ordnance that have been recovered by the ground workers on site. Providing Explosive Ordnance Safety and Awareness briefings to any staff that have not received them earlier and advise staff of the need to modify working practices to take account of the ordnance threat. Finally, to aid Incident Management which would involve liaison with the local authorities and Police should ordnance be identified and present an explosive hazard.

- *Intrusive Magnetometer Survey of all Pile locations down to a maximum bomb penetration depth:* BACTEC can deploy a range of intrusive magnetometry techniques to clear ahead of all the pile/borehole locations. The appropriate technique is governed by a number of factors, but most importantly the site's ground conditions. The appropriate survey methodology would be confirmed once the enabling works have been completed. A site meeting would be required between BACTEC and the client to determine the methodology suitable for this site.

- *Target Investigation:* Any anomalies highlighted during the intrusive survey which model as WWII-era air delivered bombs would be investigated.

Area B:

- *Explosive Ordnance Disposal (EOD) Engineer On-Call during excavations to the maximum bomb penetration depth:* When instructed, an Engineer is briefed on the Project and this UXO Threat Assessment. In the event of a suspected UXO Incident, the Engineer can be called and a fast deployment will quickly deal with the situation thereby reducing the 'down time' for the Contractor. The on-call measure would be appropriate when an EOD Engineer is not already on site.

In making this assessment and recommending the following risk mitigation measures, the proposed works outlined in the 'Scope of the Proposed Works' section were considered. However; should the planned works be changed in detail or additional intrusive engineering works be proposed, BACTEC should be consulted to re-assess the threat from explosive ordnance.

15. CONCLUSIONS

15.1. Summary

The borough of St Marylebone suffered heavy bombing raids in the early years of WWII. The site itself sustained a bomb strike in the north-west corner and it is suggested that this caused the reconstruction of 62 Marylebone High Street/13 Marylebone Road. In addition, the areas surrounding the site to the east, west, north and south all sustained bomb strikes with the closest to site being recorded on Park Crescent, Portland Place and on Harley Street. These are all within 200 metres (m) of the site. The bomb strikes on Park Crescent are approximately 100m east of the site. The area in general held strategic targets of importance for the Luftwaffe, such as the main line stations and rail marshalling yards and these were repeatedly bombed in the hope of disrupting the rail system. In addition a power station to the north-west, which was photographed by reconnaissance aircraft before the war, was targeted. There are no bomb strikes or bomb damage recorded on the London Clinic main building.

15.2. Recommendations

Taking into account the findings of this study and the known extent of the proposed works BACTEC considers that there is a **medium to high** threat from UXB in the Area A and a **low to medium** threat in Area B. Therefore the following risk mitigation measures are recommended to support the future intrusive works at The London Clinic Cancer Centre.

All Intrusive Works

- Explosive Ordnance Safety and Awareness Briefings to all personnel conducting intrusive works.

Area A

- Explosive Ordnance Disposal (EOD) Engineer Presence on Site to monitor all excavations to a maximum bomb penetration depth.
- Intrusive Magnetometer Survey of all Pile locations down to a maximum bomb penetration depth and target investigation if required.

THE LONDON CLINIC   THE LONDON CLINIC CANCER CENTRE

Area B

- Explosive Ordnance Disposal (EOD) Engineer On-Call during excavations to the maximum bomb penetration depth.

16. BIBLIOGRAPHY

The published documents consulted during this assessment are listed below.

- Clarke, N.J., *Adolf Hitler's Home Counties Holiday Snaps: German Aerial Reconnaissance Photography of London and the Home Counties 1939-1942*, Nigel J Clarke Publications. 1996.

- Fegan, T., *The Baby Killers: German Air Raids on Britain in the First World War*, Leo Cooper. 2001.

- Fleischer, W., *German Air-Dropped Weapons to 1945*, Midland Publishing. 2004.

- Ramsey, W., *The Blitz Then and Now, Volume 1*, Battle of Britain Prints International Limited. 1987.

- Ramsey, W., *The Blitz Then and Now, Volume 2*, Battle of Britain Prints International Limited. 1988.

- Ramsey, W., *The Blitz Then and Now, Volume 3*, Battle of Britain Prints International Limited. 1990.

The London Clinic Cancer Centre
EXPLOSIVE ORDNANCE THREAT ASSESSMENT REPORT

ANNEX A – SITE LOCATION MAPS

Produced by BACTEC International Limited
For The London Clinic

Reference 8936TA 06/01/06

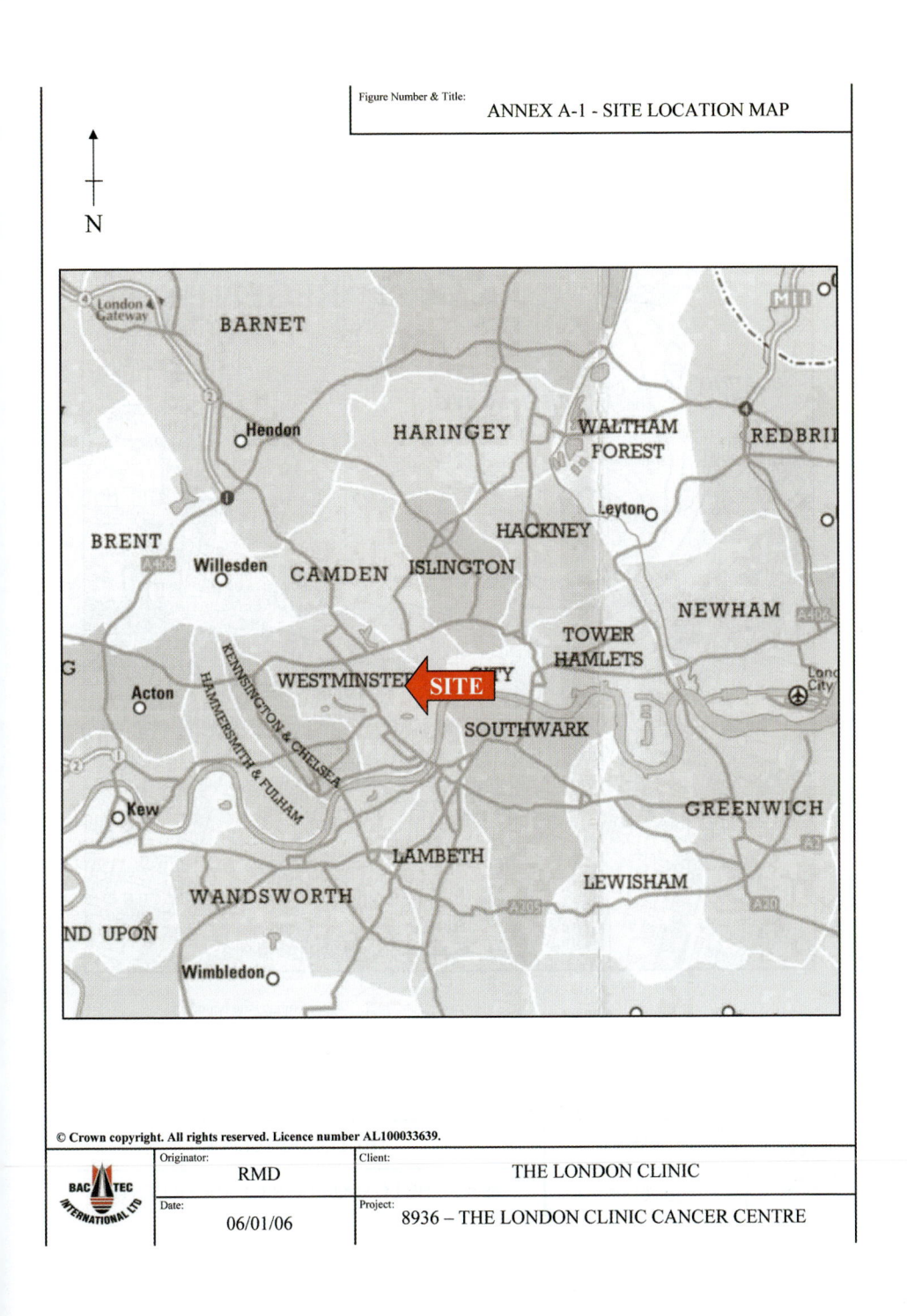

Appendix 13: Explosive ordance threat assessment etc. **213**

Figure Number & Title: ANNEX A-1 - SITE LOCATION MAP

© Crown copyright. All rights reserved. Licence number AL100033639.

Originator: RMD	Client: THE LONDON CLINIC
Date: 06/01/06	Project: 8936 – THE LONDON CLINIC CANCER CENTRE

A History of The London Clinic

Figure Number & Title: ANNEX A-2 - SITE LOCATION MAP

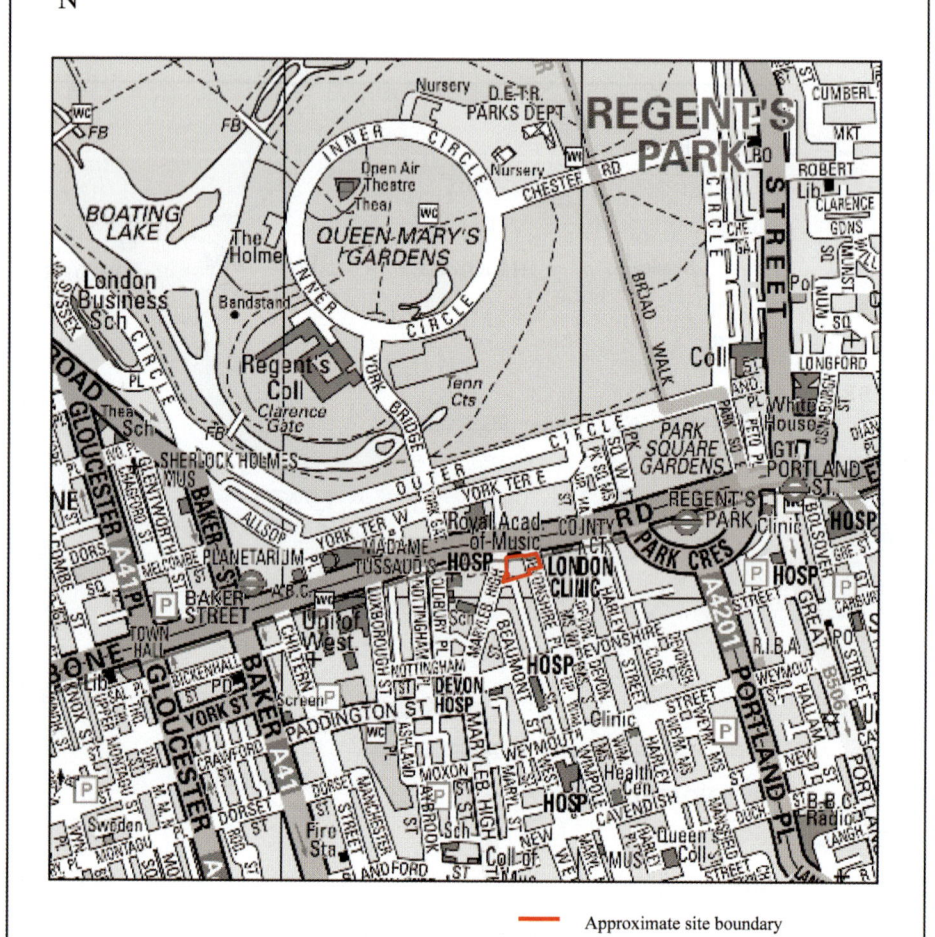

Approximate site boundary

© Crown copyright. All rights reserved. Licence number AL100033639.

	Originator: RMD	Client: THE LONDON CLINIC
BAC TEC INTERNATIONAL LTD	Date: 06/01/06	Project: 8936 – THE LONDON CLINIC CANCER CENTRE

Appendix 13: Explosive ordance threat assessment etc. **215**

The London Clinic Cancer Centre
EXPLOSIVE ORDNANCE THREAT ASSESSMENT REPORT

ANNEX B – 2003 AERIAL PHOTOGRAPH

Reproduced with permission from Getmapping plc.

Produced by BACTEC International Limited
For The London Clinic

Reference 8936TA 06/01/06

A History of The London Clinic

Figure Number & Title:
ANNEX B – 2003 AERIAL PHOTOGRAPH

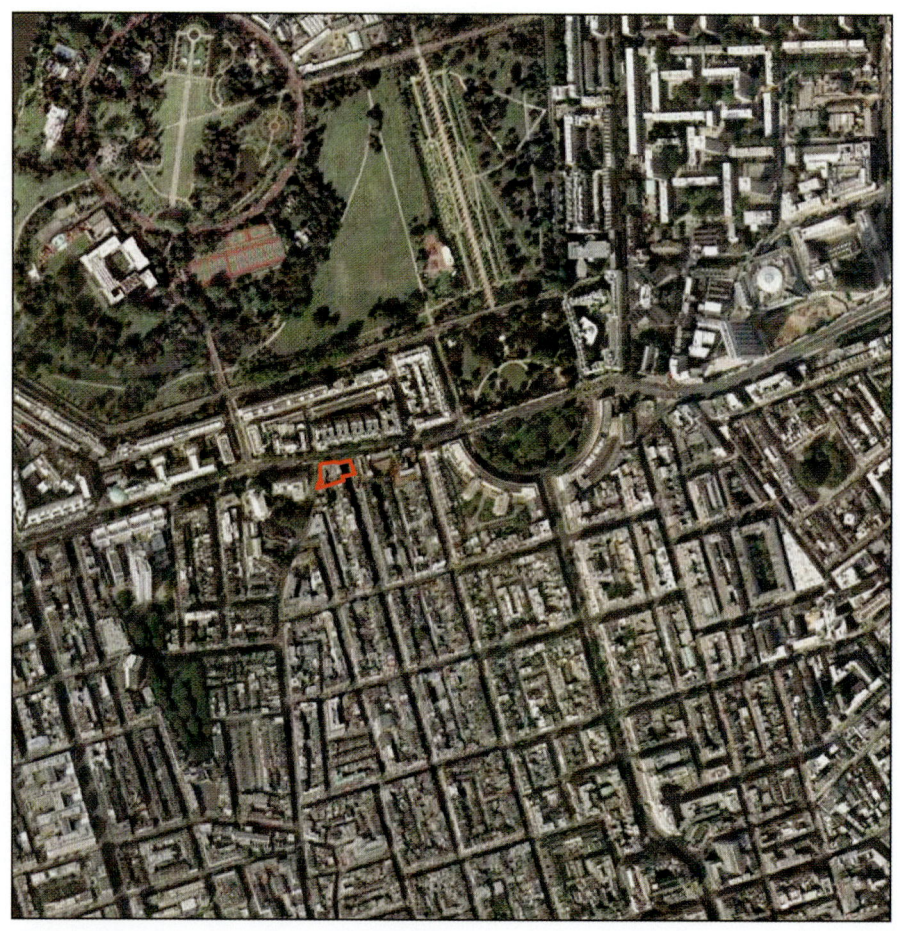

— Approximate site boundary

Source: GETMAPPING

	Originator:	Client:	
BAC TEC INTERNATIONAL LTD	RMD	THE LONDON CLINIC	
	Date: 06/01/06	Project: 8936 – THE LONDON CLINIC CANCER CENTRE	

The London Clinic Cancer Centre
EXPLOSIVE ORDNANCE THREAT ASSESSMENT REPORT

ANNEX C – SITE PLANS

Produced by BACTEC International Limited
For The London Clinic

Reference 8936TA 06/01/06

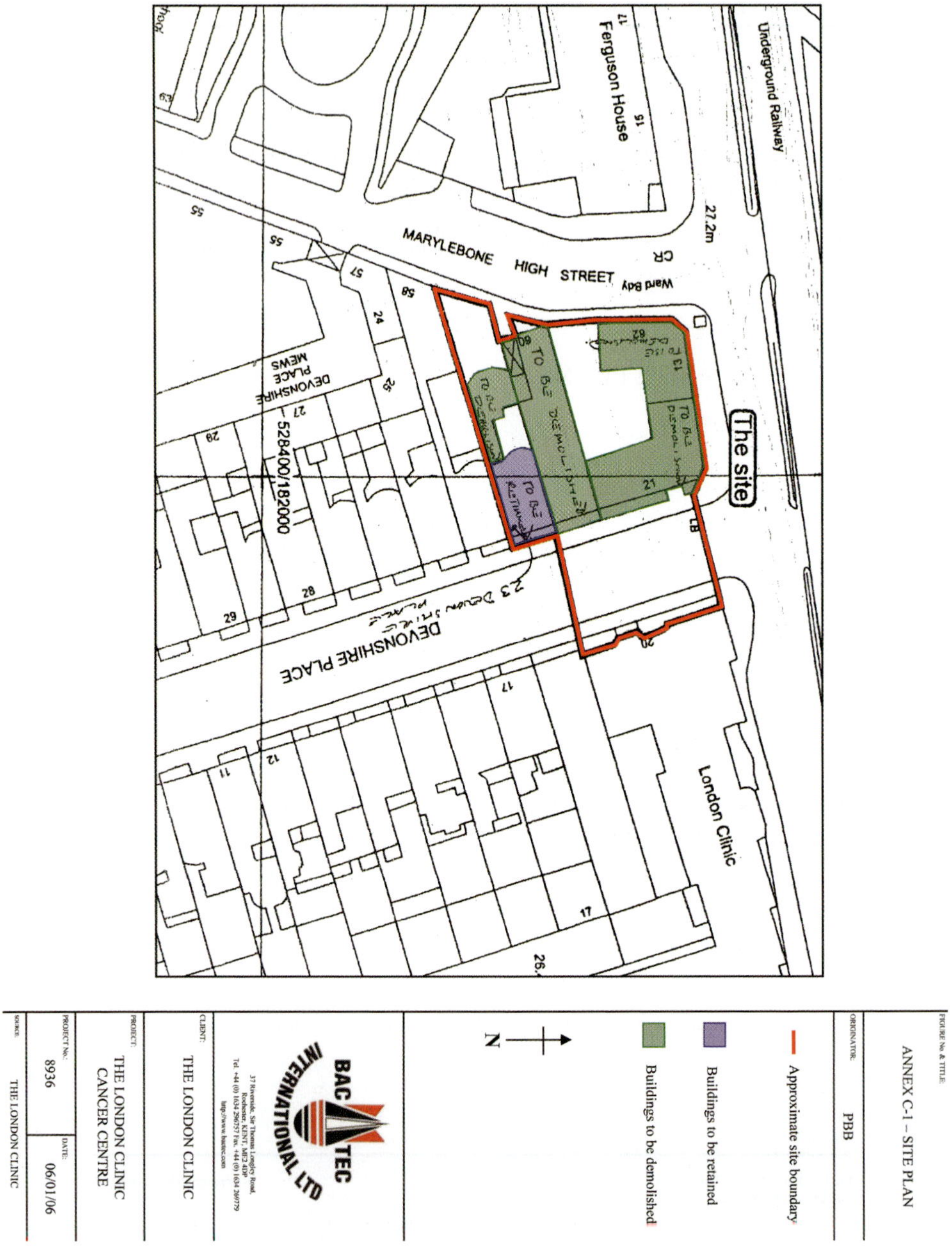
Underground Railway
Ferguson House
27.2m
MARYLEBONE HIGH STREET
The site
TO BE DEMOLISHED
TO BE RETAINED
DEVONSHIRE PLACE MEWS
528400/182000
DEVONSHIRE PLACE
London Clinic
FIGURE No. & TITLE:
ANNEX C-1 – SITE PLAN
ORIGINATOR:
PBB
Approximate site boundary
Buildings to be retained
Buildings to be demolished
N
BAC TEC INTERNATIONAL LTD
CLIENT:
THE LONDON CLINIC
PROJECT:
THE LONDON CLINIC CANCER CENTRE
PROJECT No.:
8936
DATE:
06/01/06
SOURCE:
THE LONDON CLINIC

Appendix 13: Explosive ordance threat assessment etc. **219**

ANNEX C-2 – SITE PLAN

Current buildings on site — Approximate site boundary

Source: The London Clinic

Originator:	RMD	Client:	THE LONDON CLINIC
Date:	06/01/06	Project:	8936 – THE LONDON CLINIC CANCER CENTRE

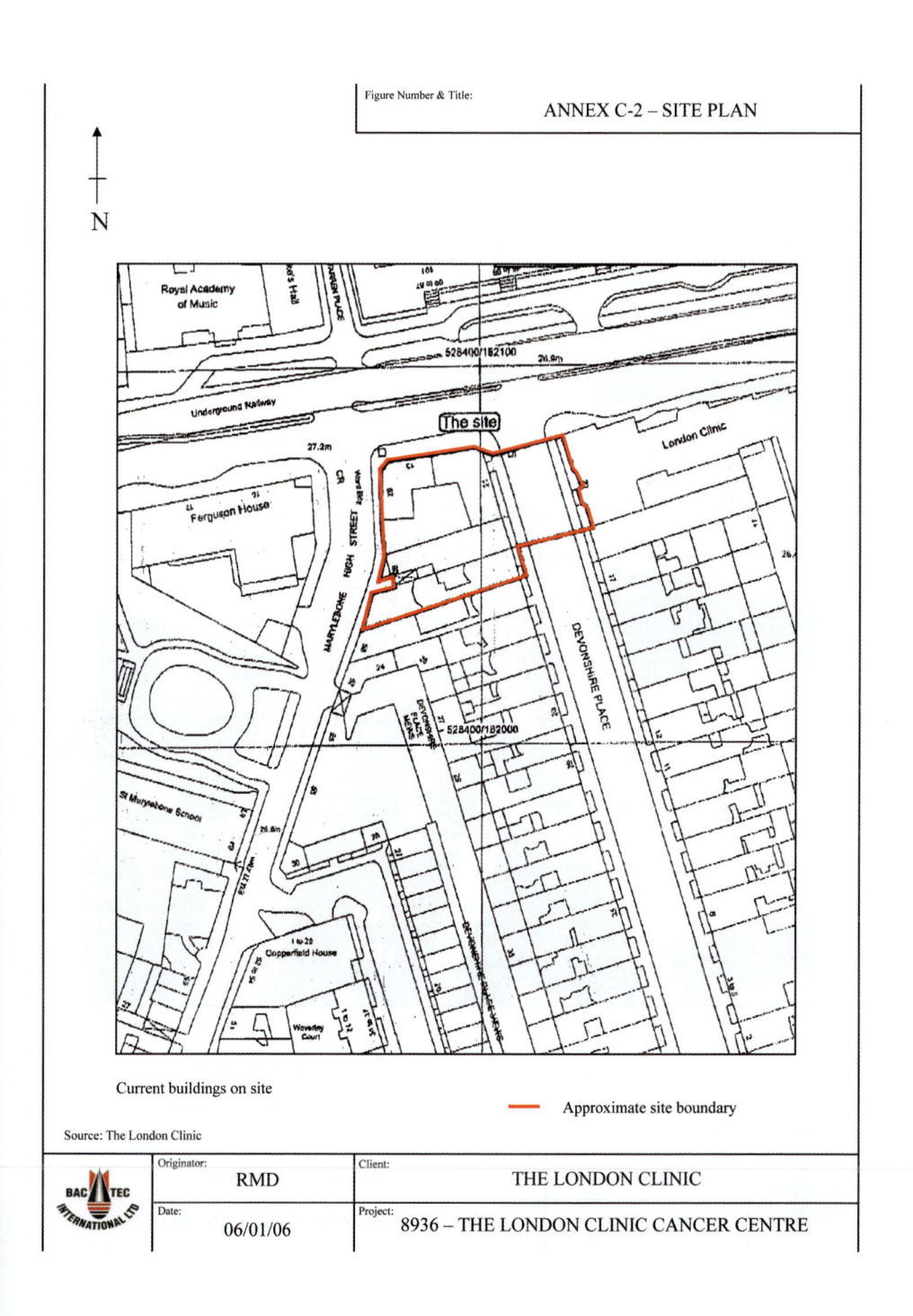

220 A History of The London Clinic

Figure Number & Title: ANNEX C-3 – SITE PLAN

Final new build perimeter

Location of link tunnel

Approximate site boundary

Source: The London Clinic

Originator:	RMD	Client:	THE LONDON CLINIC
Date:	06/01/06	Project:	8936 – THE LONDON CLINIC CANCER CENTRE

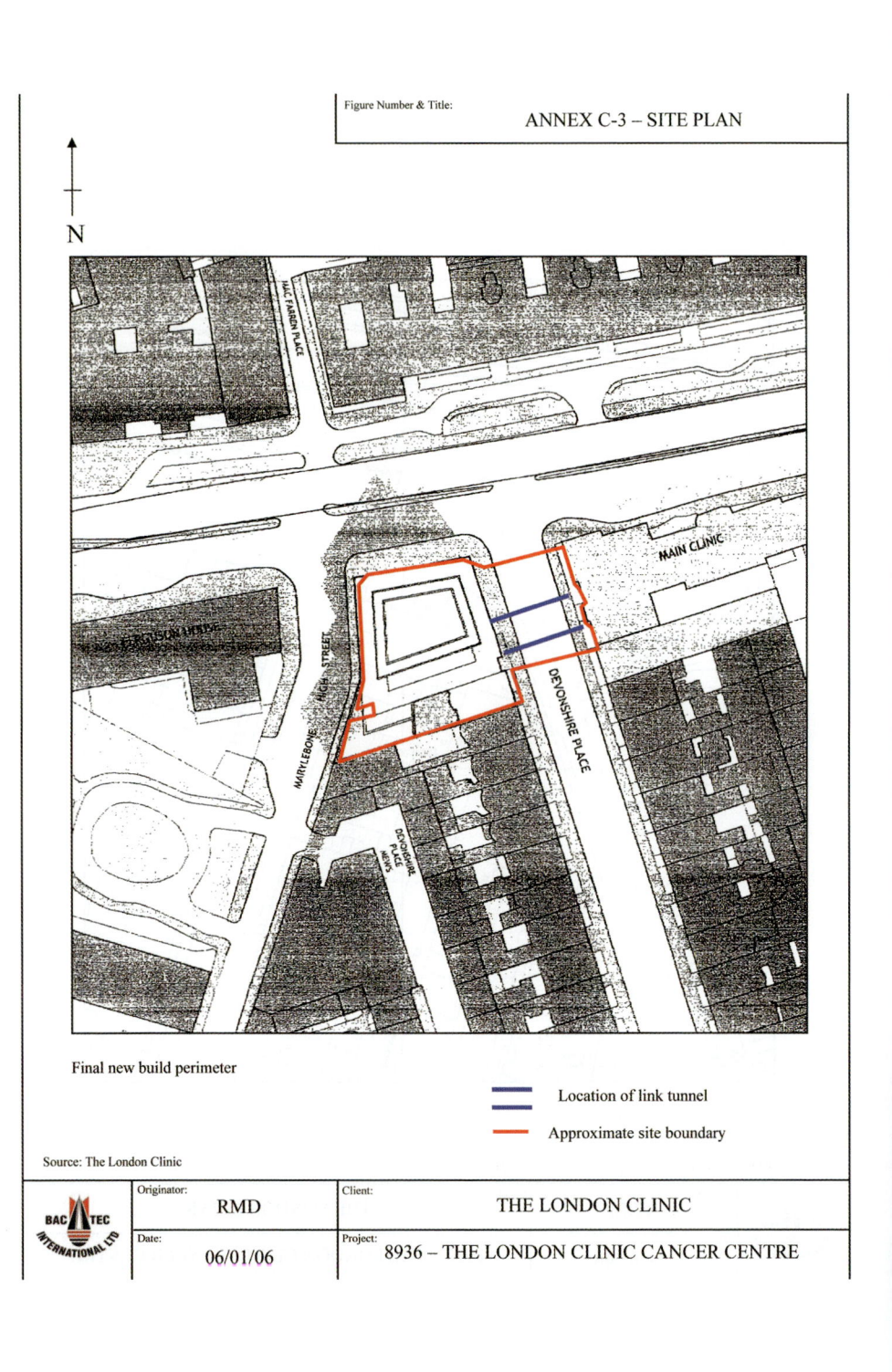

Appendix 13: Explosive ordance threat assessment etc. **221**

The London Clinic Cancer Centre
EXPLOSIVE ORDNANCE THREAT ASSESSMENT REPORT

ANNEX D – WWI BOMB PLOT OF LONDON

Reproduced with permission from The National Archives ref HO193/5.

Produced by BACTEC International Limited
For The London Clinic

Reference 8936TA 06/01/06

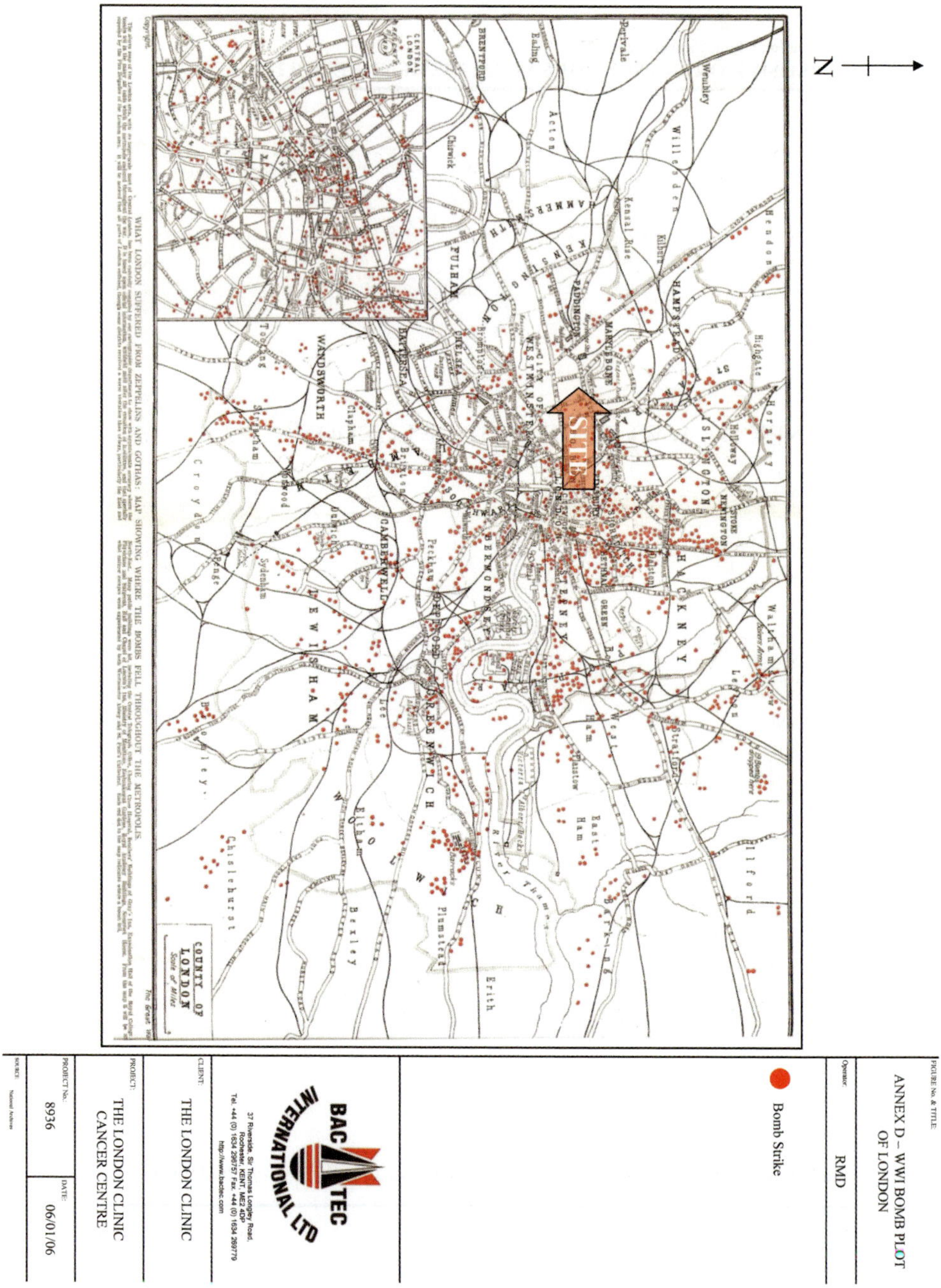
WHAT LONDON SUFFERED FROM ZEPPELINS AND GOTHAS: MAP SHOWING WHERE THE BOMBS FELL THROUGHOUT THE METROPOLIS
SITE
N
COUNTY OF LONDON
CENTRAL LONDON
FIGURE No. & TITLE:
ANNEX D – WWI BOMB PLOT OF LONDON
Operator:
RMD
Bomb Strike
BAC TEC INTERNATIONAL LTD
37 Riverside, Sir Thomas Longley Road, Rochester, KENT, ME2 4DP
Tel. +44 (0) 1634 296757 Fax. +44 (0) 1634 299779
http://www.bactec.com
CLIENT:
THE LONDON CLINIC
PROJECT:
THE LONDON CLINIC CANCER CENTRE
PROJECT No.:
8936
DATE:
06/01/06
SOURCE:
National Archives

Appendix 13: Explosive ordance threat assessment etc. **223**

The London Clinic Cancer Centre
EXPLOSIVE ORDNANCE THREAT ASSESSMENT REPORT

ANNEX E – WAR DAMAGE MAP

Reproduced with permission from The National Archives ref HO193/5.

Produced by BACTEC International Limited
For The London Clinic

Reference 8936TA 06/01/06

224   *A History of The London Clinic*

ANNEX E – WAR DAMAGE MAP

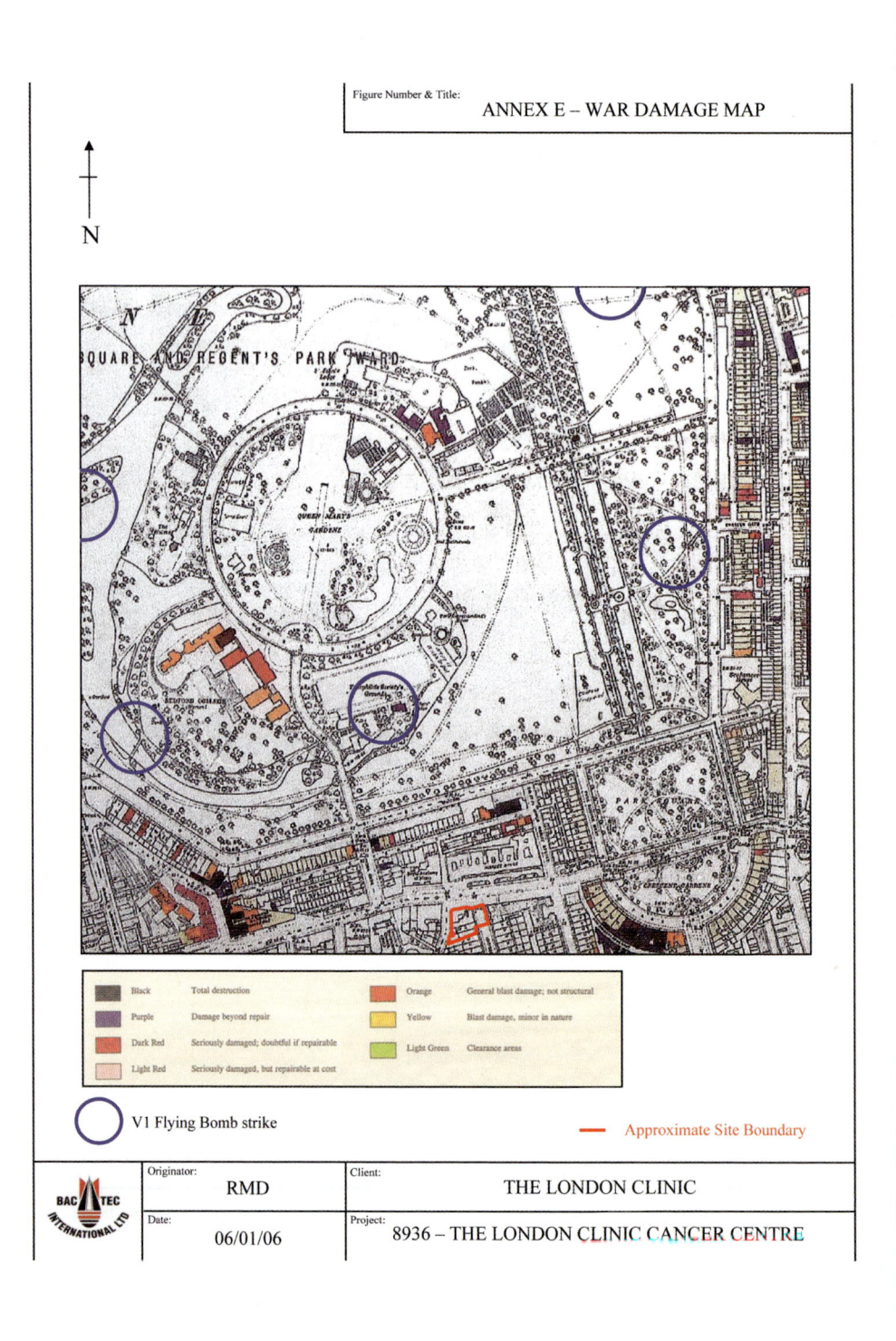

Appendix 13: Explosive ordance threat assessment etc. **225**

The London Clinic Cancer Centre
EXPLOSIVE ORDNANCE THREAT ASSESSMENT REPORT

ANNEX F – LUFTWAFFE TARGET RECONNAISSANCE
PHOTOGRAPH

Reproduced with kind permission from Nigel J Clarke publications,
www.njcpublications.co.uk

Produced by BACTEC International Limited
For The London Clinic

Reference 8936TA 06/01/06

226   *A History of The London Clinic*

Figure Number & Title:	ANNEX F – LUFTWAFFE TARGET RECONNAISSANCE PHOTOGRAPH

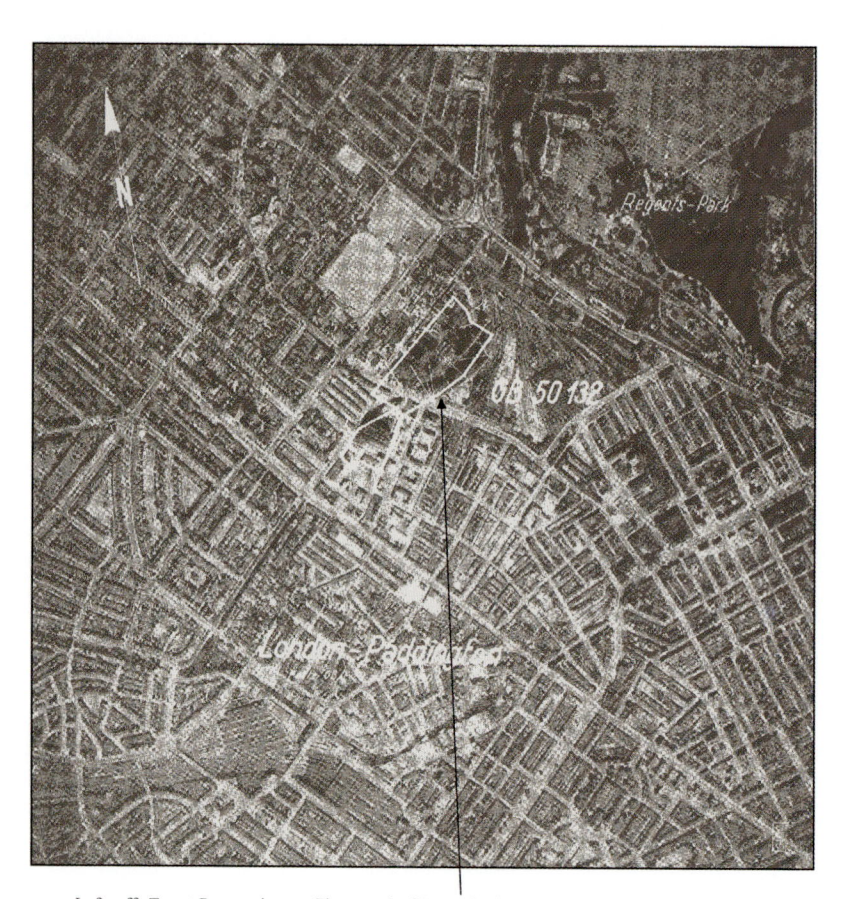

Luftwaffe Target Reconnaissance Photograph of Power Station and Marshalling Yards in Paddington

The study site is just off this photograph to the east

SOURCE: Adolf Hitler's Home Counties Holiday Snaps

	Originator:	RMD	Client:	THE LONDON CLINIC
BAC TEC INTERNATIONAL LTD	Date:	06/01/06	Project:	8936 – THE LONDON CLINIC CANCER CENTRE

Appendix 13: Explosive ordance threat assessment etc. **227**

The London Clinic Cancer Centre
EXPLOSIVE ORDNANCE THREAT ASSESSMENT REPORT

ANNEX G – BOMB DENSITY MAP

Produced by BACTEC International Limited
For The London Clinic

Reference 8936TA 06/01/06

228 *A History of The London Clinic*

Figure Number & Title: **ANNEX G – BOMB DENSITY MAP**

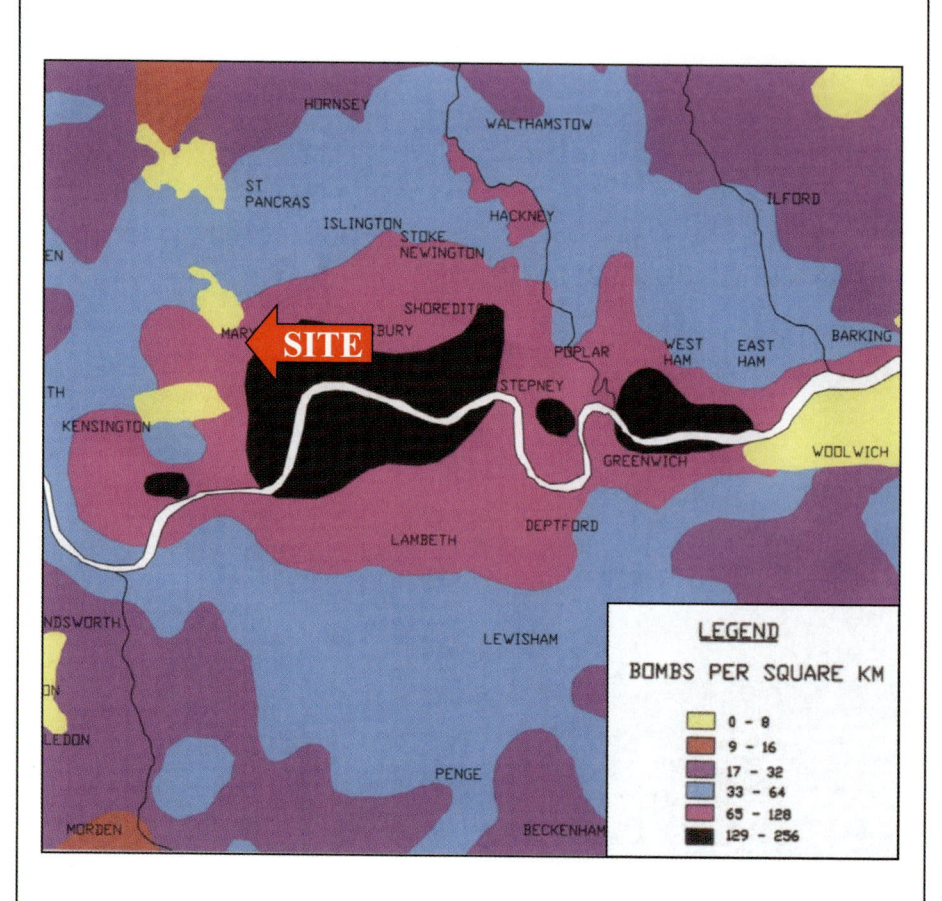

LEGEND
BOMBS PER SQUARE KM
- 0 – 8
- 9 – 16
- 17 – 32
- 33 – 64
- 65 – 128
- 129 – 256

The map depicts the density of bombs that fell on Greater London throughout the duration of WWII

Originator: RMD	Client: THE LONDON CLINIC
Date: 06/01/06	Project: 8936 – THE LONDON CLINIC CANCER CENTRE

BACTEC INTERNATIONAL LTD

Appendix 13: Explosive ordance threat assessment etc. **229**

The London Clinic Cancer Centre
EXPLOSIVE ORDNANCE THREAT ASSESSMENT REPORT

ANNEX H – BOMB CENSUS MAPS

Reproduced with permission from The National Archives ref HO193/5.

Produced by BACTEC International Limited
For The London Clinic

Reference 8936TA 06/01/06

230 A History of The London Clinic

Figure Number & Title:
ANNEX H-1 – BOMB CENSUS MAP

BOMB CENSUS MAP HO 193/4 – No Date.

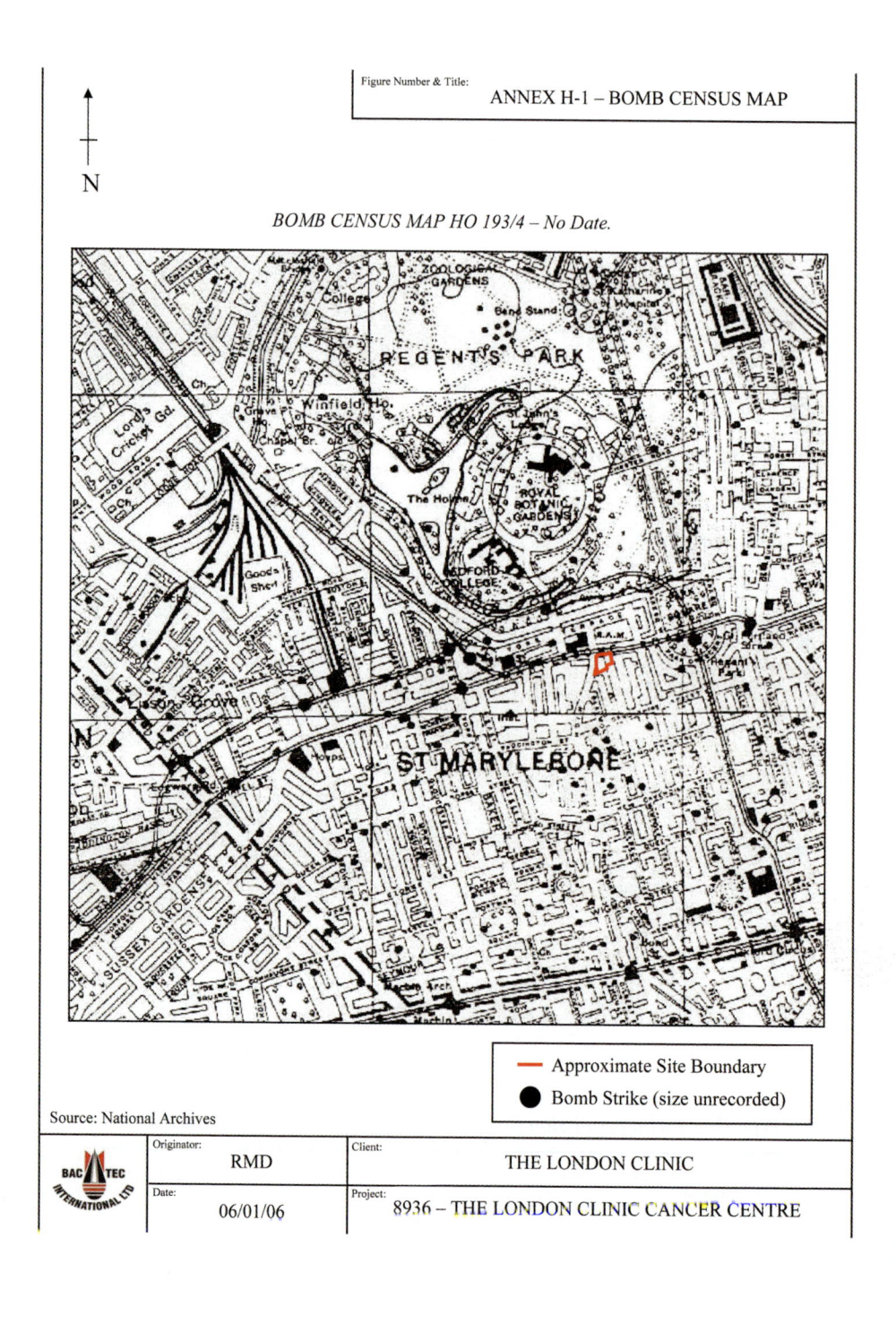

— Approximate Site Boundary
● Bomb Strike (size unrecorded)

Source: National Archives

Originator: RMD
Client: THE LONDON CLINIC
Date: 06/01/06
Project: 8936 – THE LONDON CLINIC CANCER CENTRE

Appendix 13: Explosive ordance threat assessment etc. **231**

Figure Number & Title: **ANNEX H-2 – BOMB CENSUS MAP**

BOMB CENSUS MAP HO 193/12 – Night Bombing Up to 6/7/1940

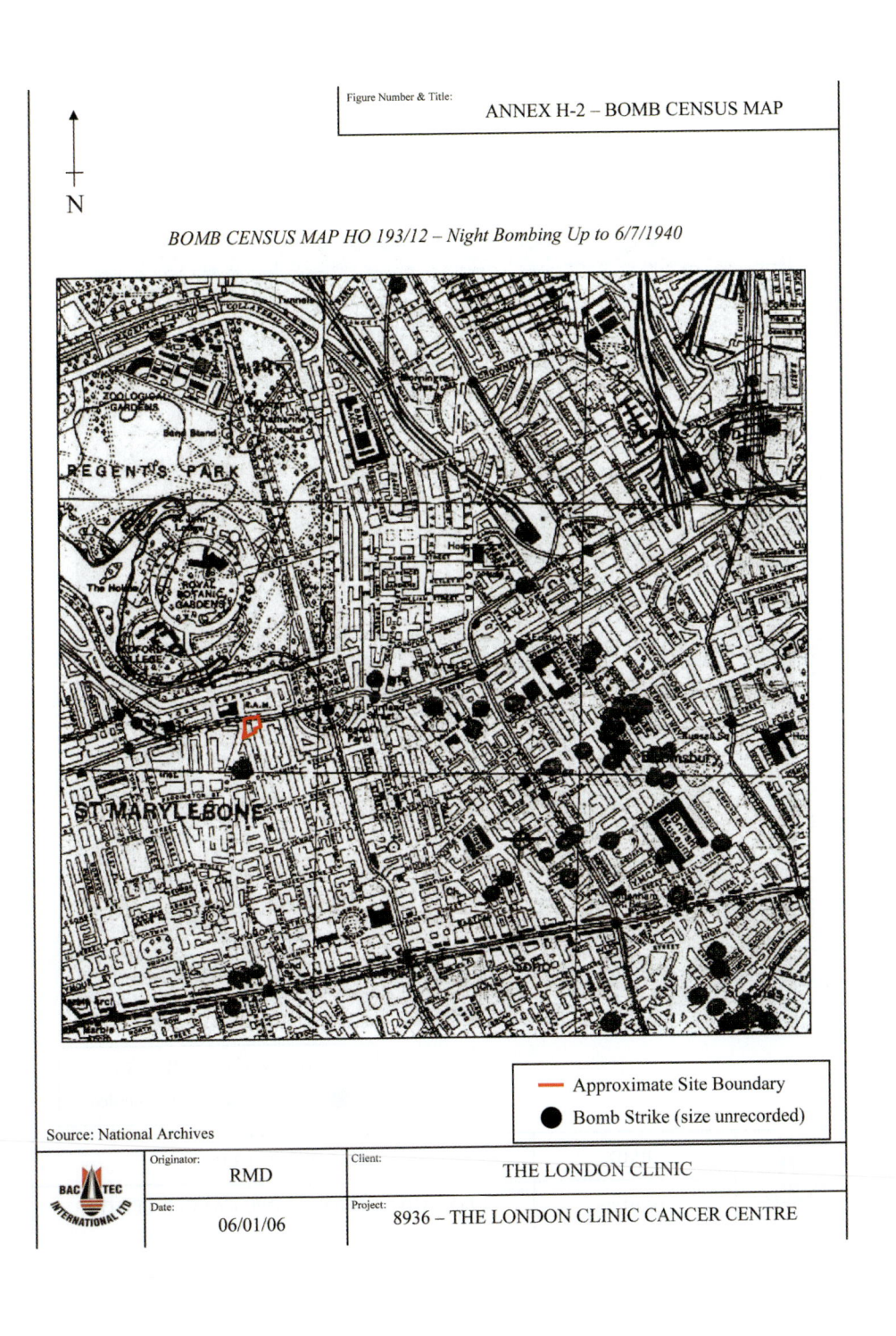

— Approximate Site Boundary
● Bomb Strike (size unrecorded)

Source: National Archives

Originator: RMD	Client: THE LONDON CLINIC
Date: 06/01/06	Project: 8936 – THE LONDON CLINIC CANCER CENTRE

232 — A History of The London Clinic

Figure Number & Title: ANNEX H-3– BOMB CENSUS MAP

BOMB CENSUS MAP HO 193/5 – 11-18/11/1940

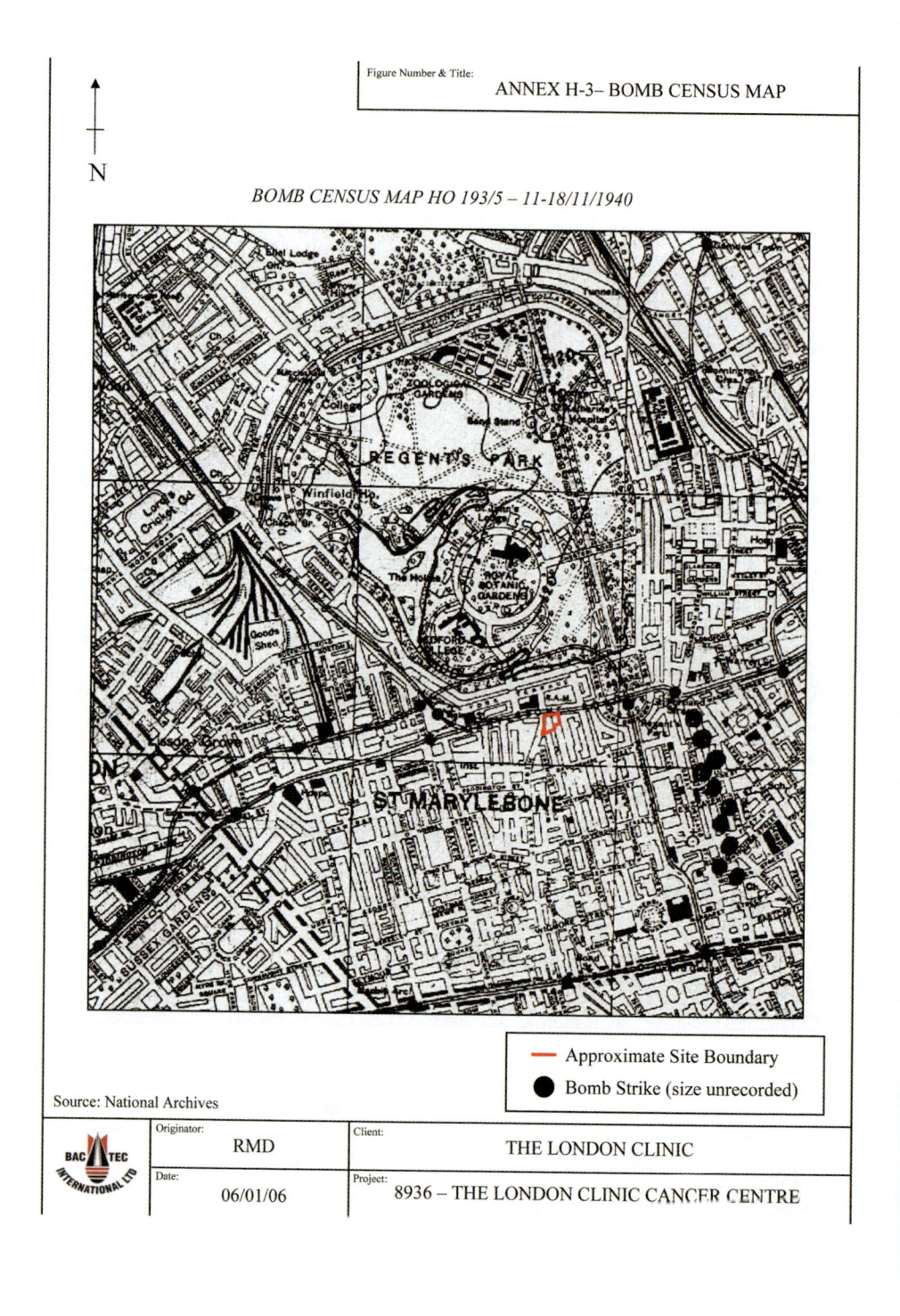

— Approximate Site Boundary
● Bomb Strike (size unrecorded)

Source: National Archives

Originator:	Client:	
BACTEC INTERNATIONAL LTD	RMD	THE LONDON CLINIC
Date: 06/01/06	Project: 8936 – THE LONDON CLINIC CANCER CENTRE	

Appendix 13: Explosive ordance threat assessment etc. **233**

Figure Number & Title: ANNEX H-4 – BOMB CENSUS MAP

BOMB CENSUS MAP HO 193/13 – 7/10/1940-6/6/1941

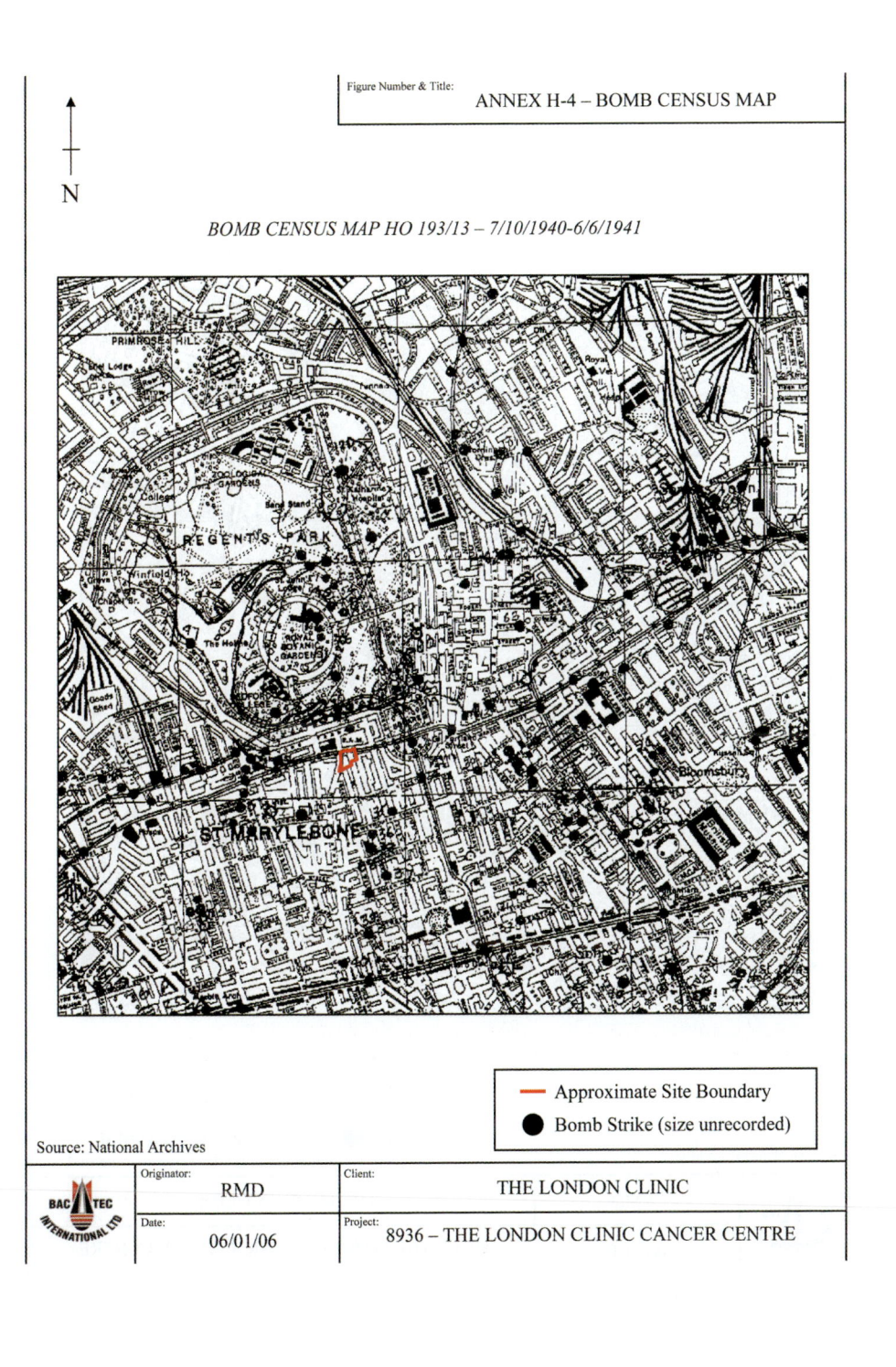

— Approximate Site Boundary
● Bomb Strike (size unrecorded)

Source: National Archives

Originator: RMD	Client: THE LONDON CLINIC
Date: 06/01/06	Project: 8936 – THE LONDON CLINIC CANCER CENTRE

Figure Number & Title: ANNEX H-5 – BOMB CENSUS MAP

BOMB CENSUS MAP HO 193/28 – 5/5/1941-12/5/1941

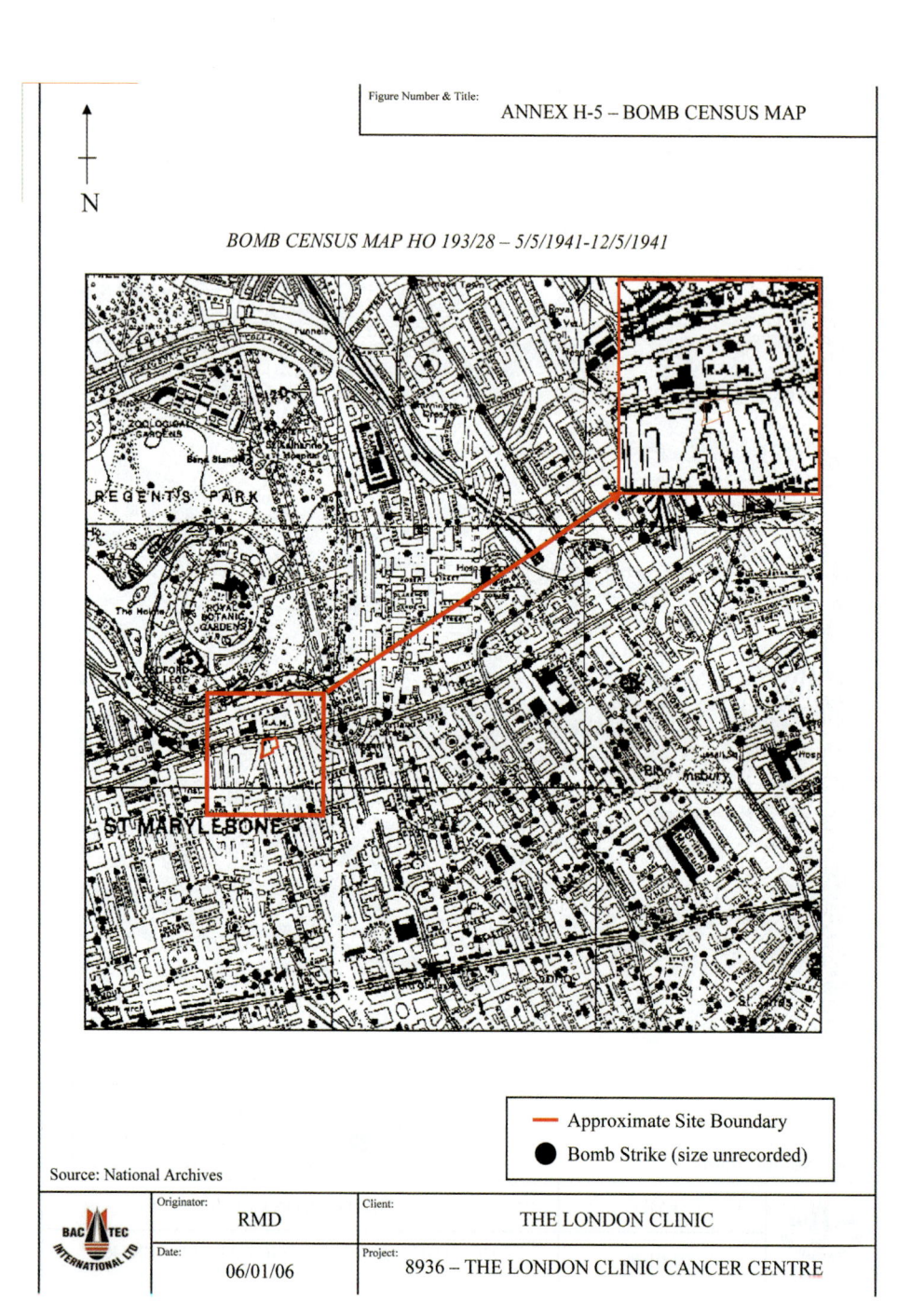

— Approximate Site Boundary
● Bomb Strike (size unrecorded)

Source: National Archives

Originator:	RMD	Client:	THE LONDON CLINIC
Date:	06/01/06	Project:	8936 – THE LONDON CLINIC CANCER CENTRE

Appendix 13: Explosive ordance threat assessment etc. **235**

The London Clinic Cancer Centre
EXPLOSIVE ORDNANCE THREAT ASSESSMENT REPORT

ANNEX I – LONDON BOMB DAMAGE PHOTOGRAPHS

Produced by BACTEC International Limited
For The London Clinic

Reference 8936TA 06/01/06

236 *A History of The London Clinic*

ANNEX I – LONDON BOMB DAMAGE PHOTOGRAPHS

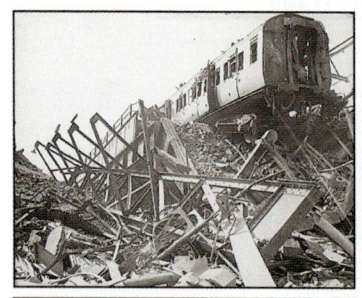

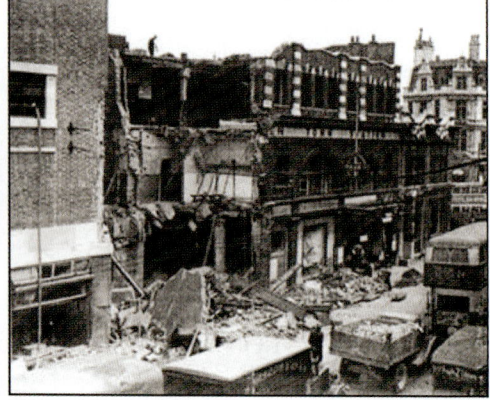

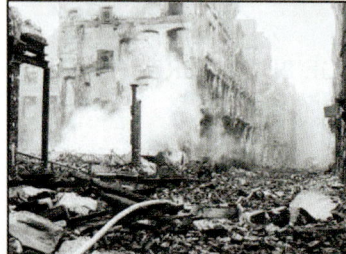

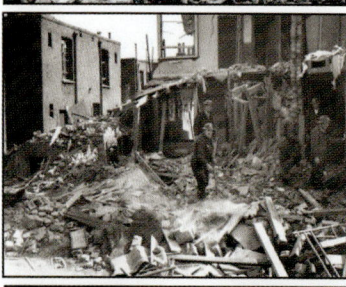

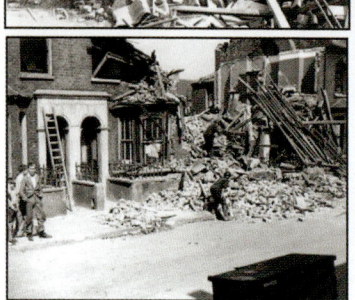

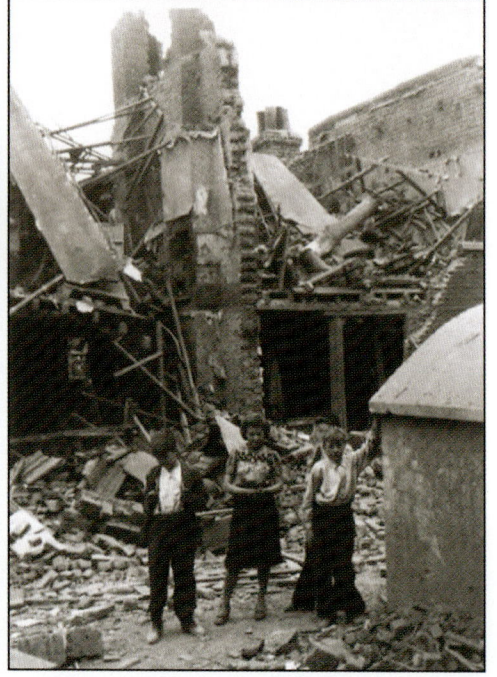

| Originator: RMD | Client: THE LONDON CLINIC |
| Date: 06/01/06 | Project: 8936 – THE LONDON CLINIC CANCER CENTRE |

Appendix 13: Explosive ordance threat assessment etc. **237**

The London Clinic Cancer Centre
EXPLOSIVE ORDNANCE THREAT ASSESSMENT REPORT

ANNEX J – GERMAN AIR-DELIVERED ORDNANCE

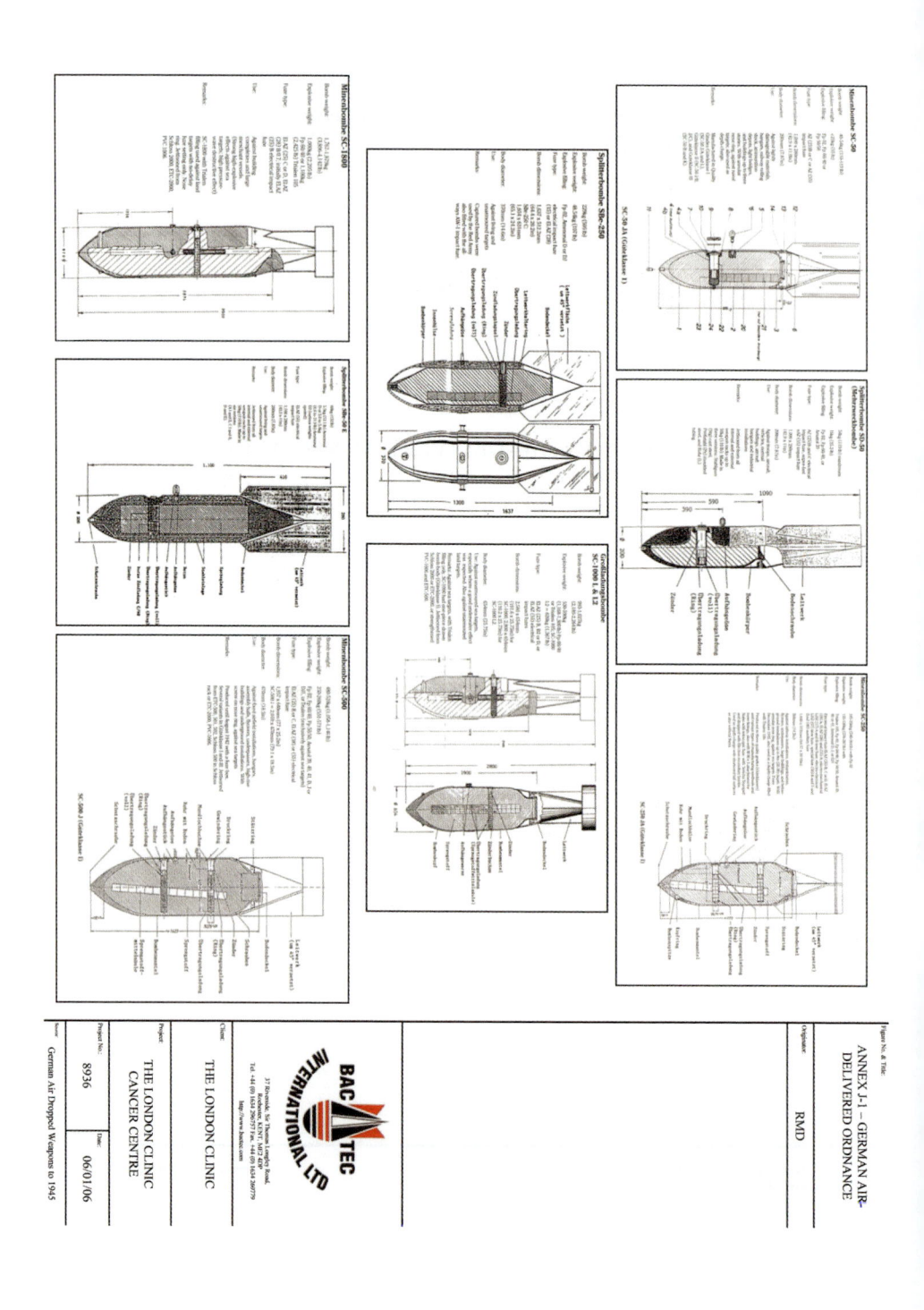

238 — A History of The London Clinic

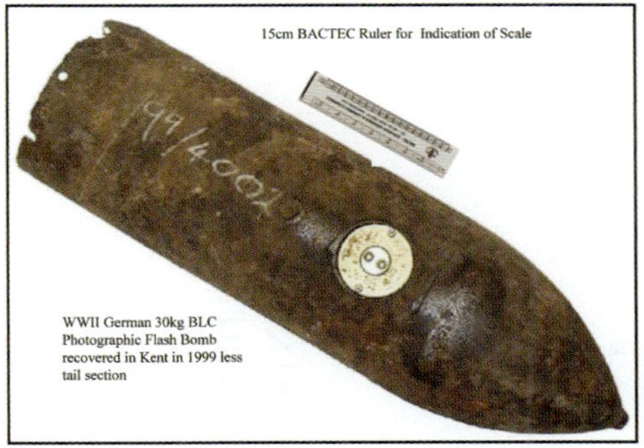

Appendix 13: Explosive ordance threat assessment etc. **239**

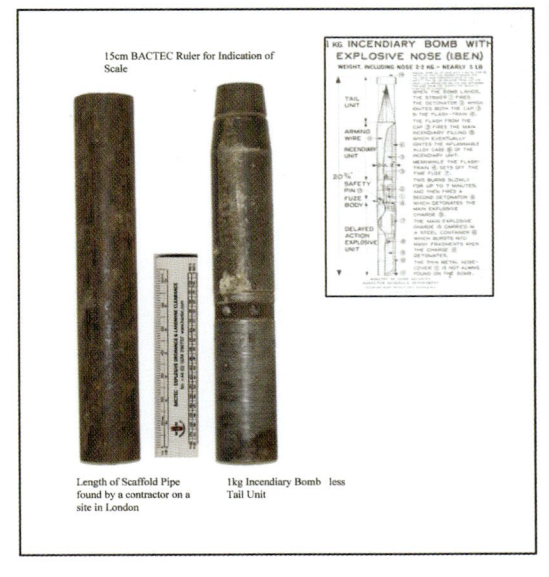

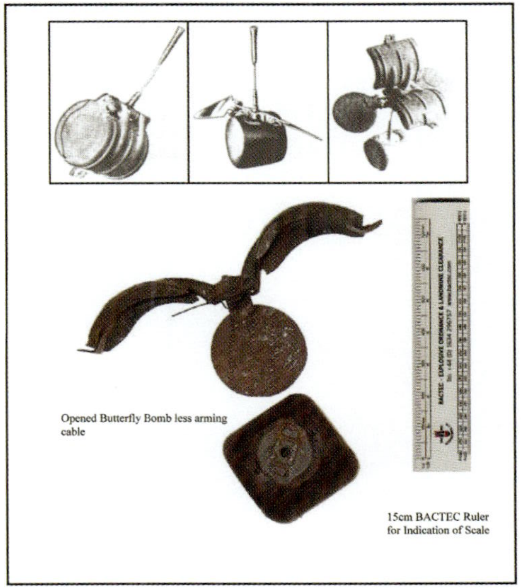

The London Clinic Cancer Centre
EXPLOSIVE ORDNANCE THREAT ASSESSMENT REPORT

ANNEX K – NEWSPAPER ARTICLE RELATING TO
                DETONATION OF A UXB DURING
                INTRUSIVE WORKS

Produced by BACTEC International Limited   Reference 8936TA 06/01/06
For The London Clinic

Appendix 13: Explosive ordance threat assessment etc.   **241**

Figure Number & Title: ANNEX K – PRESS ARTICLE RELATING TO DETONATION OF UXB DURING INTRUSIVE WORKS

International   FRIDAY, 16 SEPTEMBER, 1994 23

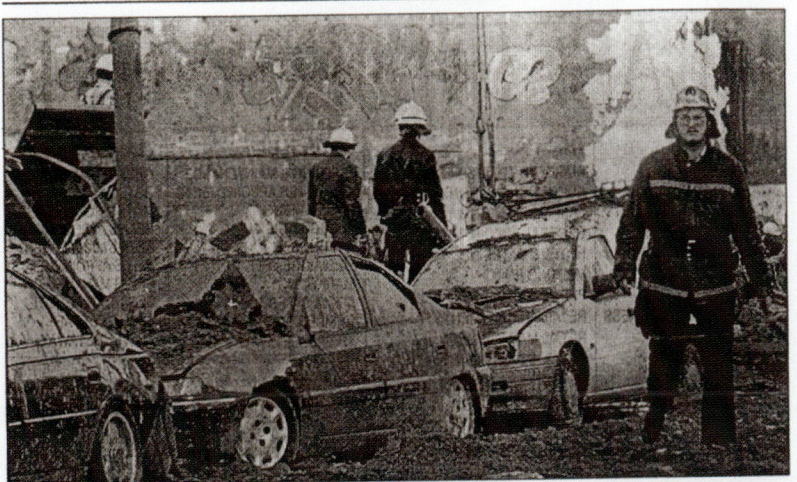

Blown up by history

RESCUE workers search for survivors after a Second World War bomb exploded at a building site in Berlin, killing three people and injuring at least eight others.

A fire brigade spokesman said he feared the final death toll could be higher. One worker was still missing, believed to be trapped under a machine. "We've found human remains 100 metres away but we can't tell if they belong to the dead already found," the spokesman said.

The blast, set off by drilling work on Frankfurter Allee, one of east Berlin's busiest avenues, trapped workers under building machinery and sent huge chunks of concrete tumbling through the air.

A large office block was being built on the site of the explosion which sent shoppers scrambling for shelter and paralysed dense afternoon traffic. One eyewitness said: "There was a bang, then silence, and then it started raining stones and dirt."

Dozens of cars within a 250-metre radius were wrecked and the top two floors of a nearby apartment block caved in. Radio reports claimed that the total number of injured stood at 14.

Originator: RMD	Client: THE LONDON CLINIC
Date: 06/01/06	Project: 8936 – THE LONDON CLINIC CANCER CENTRE

BACTEC INTERNATIONAL LTD

The London Clinic Cancer Centre
EXPLOSIVE ORDNANCE THREAT ASSESSMENT REPORT

ANNEX L – RISK MAP

Produced by BACTEC International Limited
For The London Clinic

Reference 8936TA 06/01/06

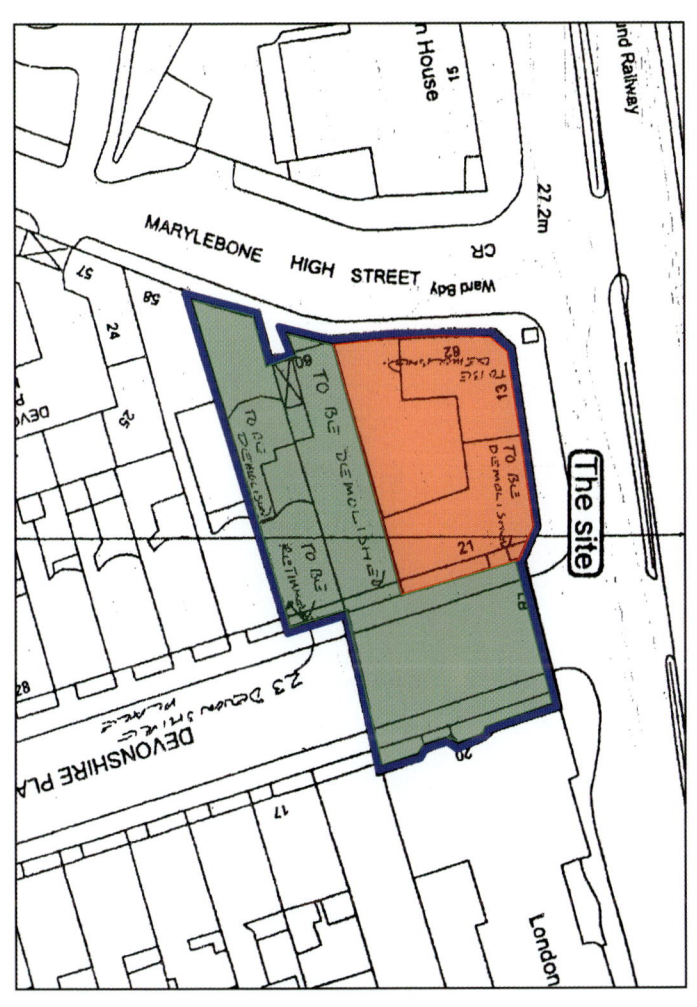

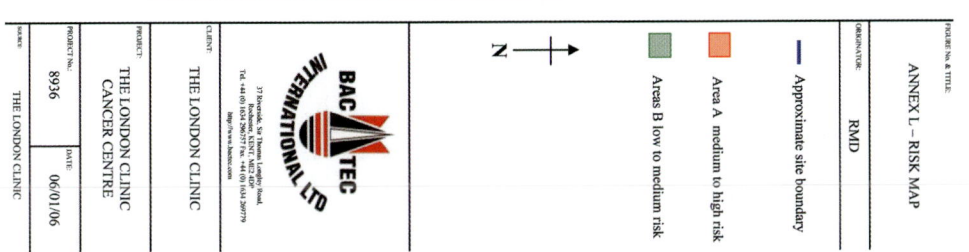

Appendix 13: Explosive ordance threat assessment etc. **243**

14
An archaeological evaluation report

(Reproduced on following pages)

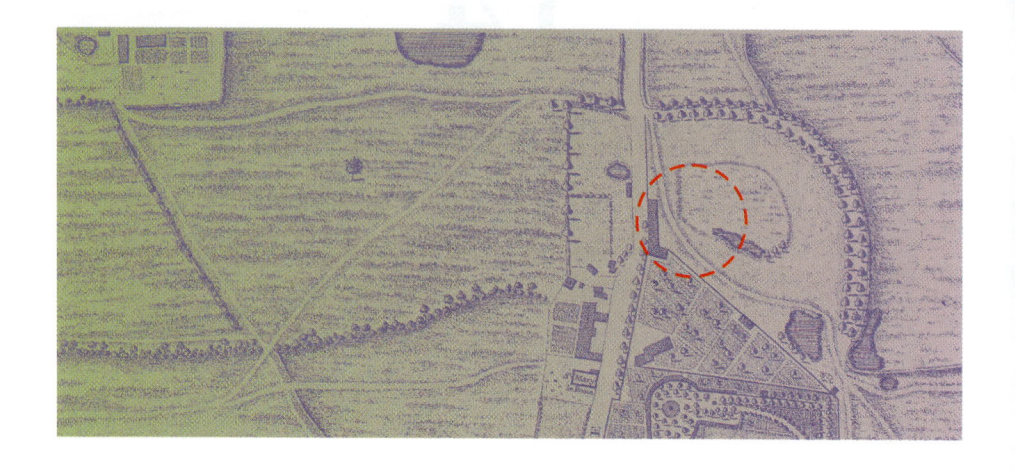

THE LONDON CANCER CLINIC
60–62 Marylebone High Street, 20–23 Devonshire Place
SE1

City of Westminster

An archaeological evaluation report

August 2006

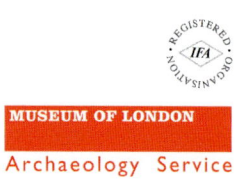

MUSEUM OF LONDON
Archaeology Service

Appendix 14: An archaeological evaluation report

THE LONDON CANCER CLINIC
60–62 Marylebone High Street,
20–23 Devonshire Place
SE1

City of Westminster

An archaeological evaluation report

Site Code: DVP06
National Grid Reference: 528390 182040

Project Manager	Rosalind Aitken
Author	Simon Gannon
Graphics	Kenneth Lymer

Museum of London Archaeology Service
© Museum of London 2006
Mortimer Wheeler House, 46 Eagle Wharf Road, London N1 7ED
tel 020 7410 2200 fax 020 7410 2201
email molas@molas.org.uk
web www.molas.org.uk

[DVP06]Evaluation report © MoLAS

Summary (non-technical)

This report presents the results of an archaeological evaluation carried out by the Museum of London Archaeology Service on the site of The London Clinic Cancer Centre, 60-62 Marylebone High Street, 20-23 Devonshire Place, London, W1. The report was commissioned from MoLAS by The London Clinic.

Following the recommendations of the previous assessment (MoLAS 2005) an evaluation trench was excavated on the site.

The results of the field evaluation have helped to refine the initial assessment of the archaeological potential of the site. Post-medieval deposits were recorded at 24.8m OD, 3.6m below the adjacent ground surface. These deposits contained substantial amounts of building material debris, likely remnants of Dove House, a 17th century Manor house. Natural sand was found at 24.8m OD.

Construction of basements within the area of the existing back garden of No. 23 Devonshire Place will remove all archaeological remains from within its footprint, including any below ground remains associated with Dove House. However the results of this evaluation have indicated that standing structural remains of Dove House are unlikely to have survived demolition.

In the light of revised understanding of the archaeological potential of the site the Museum of London Archaeology Service considers that the remaining archaeological deposits should be excavated archaeologically (ie preservation by record) under Watching Brief conditions during future ground reduction.

Appendix 14: An archaeological evaluation report

Contents

1	**Introduction**	**5**
1.1	Site background	5
1.2	Planning and legislative framework	6
1.3	Planning background	6
1.4	Origin and scope of the report	6
1.5	Aims and objectives	6
2	**Topographical and historical background**	**8**
2.1	Topography	8
2.2	Prehistoric	8
2.3	Roman	8
2.4	Saxon	8
2.5	Medieval	8
2.6	Post-medieval	9
3	**The evaluation**	**9**
3.1	Methodology	9
3.2	Results of the evaluation	11
3.3	Assessment of the evaluation	12
4	**Archaeological potential**	**13**
4.1	Realisation of original research aims	13
4.2	General discussion of potential	13
4.3	Significance	14
5	**Proposed development impact and recommendations**	**15**
6	**Acknowledgements**	**16**

[DVP06] Evaluation Report © MoLAS

7 Bibliography   **16**

8 NMR OASIS archaeological report form   **18**

   8.1 OASIS ID: molas1-17063   **18**

Appendix 14: An archaeological evaluation report **251**

[DVP06] Evaluation Report © MoLAS

List Of Illustrations

Front cover: Detail from Rocque's map of 1746
Fig 1 Site location — 21
Fig 2 Location of evaluation trench — 22
Fig 3 South facing section of evaluation trench — 23

[DVP06] Evaluation Report © MoLAS

1 Introduction

1.1 Site background

The evaluation took place in the rear garden of number 23 Devonshire Place at The London Clinic Cancer Centre, 60-62 Marylebone High Street, 20-23 Devonshire Place, London, W1, hereafter called 'the site'. It is located bounded by Marylebone High Street on the west, Marylebone Road on the north and Devonshire Place to the east. The OS National Grid Ref. for centre of site is 528390 182040. The level of the ground in the garden of 23 Devonshire Place was at 27.60m OD. The site code is DVP06.

A desk-top *Archaeological assessment (MoLAS, 2005)* and *Method Statement* (MoLAS, 2006a) were previously prepared, covering the whole area of the site. These documents should be referred to for information on the natural geology, archaeological and historical background of the site, and the initial interpretation of its archaeological potential.

An archaeological field evaluation in garden of No 23 Devonshire Place was subsequently carried out between the 10th and 13th of July 2006.

Appendix 14: An archaeological evaluation report 253

[DVP06] Evaluation Report © MoLAS

1.2 Planning and legislative framework

The legislative and planning framework in which the archaeological exercise took place was summarised in the *Method Statement* which formed the project design for the evaluation (see Section 1.2, MoLAS, 2006a).

1.3 Planning background

The evaluation was undertaken in response to a condition placed on planning permission by the local planning authority (PT/06/01023/FULL).

1.4 Origin and scope of the report

This report was commissioned by Allan Pennie on behalf of the London Clinic and produced by the Museum of London Archaeology Service (MoLAS). The report has been prepared within the terms of the relevant Standard specified by the Institute of Field Archaeologists (IFA, 2001).

Field evaluation, and the *Evaluation report* which comments on the results of that exercise, are defined in the most recent English Heritage guidelines (English Heritage, 1998) as intended to provide information about the archaeological resource in order to contribute to the:

- formulation of a strategy for the preservation or management of those remains; and/or
- formulation of an appropriate response or mitigation strategy to planning applications or other proposals which may adversely affect such archaeological remains, or enhance them; and/or
- formulation of a proposal for further archaeological investigations within a programme of research

1.5 Aims and objectives

All research is undertaken within the priorities established in the Museum of London's *A research framework for London Archaeology*, 2002

The following research aims and objectives were established in the *Method Statement* for the evaluation (Section 2.2):

- What is the nature and level of natural topography?
- What are the earliest deposits identified?
- Is there any evidence for the 17th century Dove House, in the back garden area of No 23 Devonshire Place?

- What are the latest deposits identified?

Appendix 14: An archaeological evaluation report

[DVP06] Evaluation Report © MoLAS

2 Topographical and historical background

2.1 Topography

The underlying geology of the area has been confirmed by boreholes and the archaeological evaluation of No 55–57 Marylebone High Street in 1989–90. London Clay was recorded at 7.3m below modern ground level, rising slightly from the south towards the north, up to 6.3m. Taplow Gravel overlies London Clay in this area, about 4m thick with a maximum height recorded at 24.65m OD. The top of the gravel also rises to the north, like the underlying London Clay. Up to 1m of overlying clayey silts (brickearth) was recorded at 25.35m OD with its upper surface possibly truncated by later activity. The boreholes showed that made ground (archaeological strata) was between 1.8m and 2.5m deep. To the southwest at the Marylebone School recent archaeological excavations recorded the highest level of truncated natural (brickearth over compact gravel and sand) at approximately 25.15m OD within the church.

2.2 Prehistoric

Although the Tyburn valley, with its streams and water meadows, should have provided an attractive location for both hunter-gatherer communities and the first farmers there is no evidence for *in situ* settlement from the prehistoric period in the vicinity of the site.

2.3 Roman

The 500m-wide study area around the site contains only one known find spot dated to this period. A Roman coin and bronze key found near Marylebone High Street. This lack of finds suggests a low level of activity possibly indicative of a rural environment.

2.4 Saxon

The main Middle Saxon settlement of Lundenwic was located in the area of present day Covent Garden and the Strand, *c* 2.5km to the southeast of the site. The site and surrounding area probably lay within open fields or may have been wooded. There are no known sites or finds dated to the Saxon period in the study area.

2.5 Medieval

In 1313, Marylebone manor (estate) comprised a capital message, 120 acres of arable, five acres of meadow, two acres of pasture, and a number of tenants. The original manor house was probably located near Tyburn Bridge on Oxford Street. In the eighteenth century the site was on the outskirts immediately north of this settlement.

[DVP06] Evaluation Report © MoLAS

The main Marylebone Road to the north with which the High Street now connects, was built in 1757, there is little further available information on the late medieval village.

2.6 Post-medieval

An estate plan drawn up by the Duke of Newcastle in 1708 shows the site on the very northern edge of the village of Marylebone within an open field named Dove House Park. The park is partly enclosed on its north and east sides by a line of trees. The map shows a large L-shaped building, presumably Dove House, fronting the High Street in the southwest corner of the park. The site appears to have been located within the open land to the east of the house.

Rocque's map of 1746 shows the avenue of trees that enclosed Dove House Park. The site is located in an open area to the north of a pond or ornamental lake. A footpath ran northwest–southeast across the southern part of the site.

Devonshire Place was laid out in the 1790s. Many of the original houses still stand and form part of the Harley Street Conservation Area.

Horwood's map shows that the northern side of the site, fronting onto Marylebone Road, appear had been laid out as a formal garden. The eastern side of the site, at the junction of Harley Street (then known as Ulster Street) and Marylebone Road, had been divided into building plots, prior to the houses being constructed.

By the latter half of the 19th century the formal garden on the north side of the site had been extended across the northern area and houses had been built between Devonshire Mews and Harley Street.

3 The evaluation

3.1 Methodology

All archaeological excavation and monitoring during the evaluation was carried out in accordance with the preceding *Method Statement* (MoLAS, 2006a), and the MoLAS *Archaeological Site Manual* (MoLAS, 1994).

One evaluation trench was excavated at the western limits of the rear garden of 23 Devonshire Place.

The ground was broken out and cleared by contractors under MoLAS supervision. The trench was excavated by machine by the contractors, and monitored by a member of staff from MoLAS.

Appendix 14: An archaeological evaluation report   **257**

[DVP06] Evaluation Report © MoLAS

The location of the evaluation trench was recorded by MoLAS by offsetting from adjacent standing walls and plotted on to a site plan. This information was then plotted onto the OS grid.

A written and drawn record of all archaeological deposits encountered was made in accordance with the principles set out in the MoLAS site recording manual (MoLAS, 1994). Levels were calculated from the known OD ground level.

The site has produced a trench location plan; context records; two section drawings at 1:10; and a series of digital photographs. In addition 1 box of finds were recovered from the site.

The site finds and records can be found under the site code DVP06 in the MoL archive.

[DVP06] Evaluation Report © MoLAS

3.2 Results of the evaluation

For trench locations see Fig 2

Evaluation Trench	
Location	Rear garden of 23 Devonshire Place
Dimensions	3m by 3m by 3.6m deep
Modern ground level	27.6m OD
Base of modern fill/slab	27.2m OD
Depth of archaeological deposits seen	2.4m
Level of base of deposits observed	24 m OD
Natural observed	24.8m OD

The evaluation trench was located in the rear garden of 23 Devonshire Place and measures 3m by 3m at the base.

Natural silty sands were recorded at a depth of 2.8m (24.8m OD). Overlying this was a light brown sandy silt deposit measuring 0.46m thick (context [22]) which contained occasional fragments of CBM, mortar flecks and small to medium sized pebbles. The brick samples taken have a distinctive sandy fabric (type 3065) dating to from around the mid 16th to the mid 17th century. These sandy bricks are certainly pre-Great Fire of 1666. At Rotherhithe similar sandy bricks were found in 17th century delftware waster dumps (MoLAS, 2006b). This places the deposit as contemporary with Dove House and it may represent open land/parkland.

Cut into this was a possible pit (context [21]), though only a small extent was revealed in the southeast corner of the trench. This contained a significant amount of building rubble and roofing tile, similar to that seen during the watching brief on previous geotechnical pits in the garden of No 23 (MoLAS 2006a). These fragments date to the pre-1666 fire, they can only be given an approximate date of 1450-1666, although it is more likely to be 16th or 17th century (MoLAS, 2006b). This is though to be demolition debris, possibly from the remains of Dove House, though to have been present in this area in the 17th century.

Sealing this demolition debris was a series of garden deposits dating to the 19th century.

Sealing the above deposits was a 0.40m thick layer of modern garden soil, truncated by the cut for drainage leading from No 23 Devonshire Place.

[DVP06] Evaluation Report © MoLAS

3.3 Assessment of the evaluation

GLAAS guidelines (English Heritage, 1998) require an assessment of the success of the evaluation 'in order to illustrate what level of confidence can be placed on the information which will provide the basis of the mitigation strategy'.

The trench was located in to the far south west of the site where Dove House may have stood in an area thought to be untruncated by basements.

The evaluation trench revealed several dumped deposits of post medieval date and earlier building debris probably associated with the demolition of Dove House.

A full sequence of deposits from modern deposits at ground level to natural deposits at the base of the trench was achieved.

The results concur with those derived from the archaeological monitoring of previously undertaken geotechnical works within the application site.

[DVP06] Evaluation Report © MoLAS

4 Archaeological potential

4.1 Realisation of original research aims

- What is the nature and level of natural topography?

    Natural silty sand was recorded at 24.80m OD, basements adjacent to the area of the watching brief have truncated natural deposits to a depth of *c.* 23.60m OD.

- What are the earliest deposits identified?

    The earliest deposit identified is the sandy silt deposit [22] and based on the Ceramic building material is contemporary with Dove House.
    Demolition debris found in the southeast corner of the trench also dated to 17th century (pre-fire of London). However, this demolition is likely to have occurred in the late 18th Century during the construction of the current buildings along Devonshire Place.

- Is there any evidence for the 17th century Dove House, in the back garden area of No 23 Devonshire Place?

    The survival of demolition deposits containing building debris dated to the 17th centuries may be derived from Dove House. There were no structural remains present.

- What are the latest archaeological deposits identified?

    The latest deposits identified are the 19th century garden soil deposits.

4.2 General discussion of potential

The evaluation has shown that the potential for survival of ancient ground surfaces (horizontal archaeological stratification) on the site is limited to the 17th century worked deposit representing open land/parkland. Whilst 17th century demolition debris was present on the site it is unlikely that any structural remains of Dove House are present on the site. The majority of the deposits present represent late 18th and 19th century dumped deposits and garden deposits associated with the properties fronting on to Devonshire Place.

[DVP06] Evaluation Report © MoLAS

4.3 Significance

The archaeological remains are of local significance and there is nothing to suggest that they are of regional or national importance.

[DVP06] Evaluation Report © MoLAS

5 Proposed development impact and recommendations

Construction of basements within the area of the existing back garden of No. 23 Devonshire Place would remove all archaeological remains from within its footprint, including any below ground remains associated with Dove House. However the results of this evaluation have indicated that standing structural remains of Dove House are unlikely to have survived demolition.

The Museum of London Archaeology Service considers that the remaining archaeological deposits should be excavated archaeologically excavated archaeologically (ie preservation by record) under Watching Brief conditions during future ground reduction.

The decision on the appropriate archaeological response to the deposits revealed within the evaluation trench rests with the Local Planning Authority and their designated archaeological advisor.

Appendix 14: An archaeological evaluation report 263

[DVP06] Evaluation Report © MoLAS

6 Acknowledgements

The author would like to thank the London Clinic for commissioning the work, and Alan Pennie for all his help. Thanks also to Sian Anthony (MoLAS) and Ian Betts (MoLSS) for providing his expertise on the brick samples.

7 Bibliography

ACAO, 1993 *Model briefs and specifications for archaeological assessments and field evaluations*, Association of County Archaeological Officers

BADLG, 1986 *Code of Practice, British Archaeologists and Developers Liaison Group*

City of Westminster 2002 *Unitary Development Plan*

Corporation of London Department of Planning and Transportation, 2004 *Planning Advice Note 3: Archaeology in the City of London, Archaeology Guidance*, London

Cultural Heritage Committee of the Council of Europe, 2000 *Code of Good Practice On Archaeological Heritage in Urban Development Policies; adopted at the 15th plenary session in Strasbourg on 8-10 March 2000* (CC-PAT [99] 18 rev 3)

Department of the Environment, 1990 *Planning Policy Guidance 16, Archaeology and Planning*

English Heritage, 1991 *Exploring Our Past, Strategies for the Archaeology of England*

English Heritage, May 1998 *Capital Archaeology. Strategies for sustaining the historic legacy of a world city*

English Heritage, 1991 *Management of Archaeological Projects (MAP2)*

English Heritage Greater London Archaeology Advisory Service, June 1998 *Archaeological Guidance Papers 1-5*

English Heritage Greater London Archaeology Advisory Service, May 1999 *Archaeological Guidance Papers 6*

Institute of Field Archaeologists, (IFA), 2001 *By-Laws, Standards and Policy Statements of the Institute of Field Archaeologists, (*rev. 2001), *Standard and guidance: field evaluation*

[DVP06] Evaluation Report © MoLAS

Institute of Field Archaeologists (IFA), supplement 2001, *By-Laws, Standards and Policy Statements of the Institute of Field Archaeologists: Standards and guidance – the collection, documentation conservation and research of archaeological materials*

MoLAS 2005, *21-23 Devonshire Place: Archaeological impact assessment.* unpub client report

MoLAS 2006a, the London Clinic Cancer Centre 60-62 Marylebone High Street, *21-23 Devonshire Place: Method Statement for an archaeological evaluation and watching brief,* unpub. rep.

MoLAS, 2006b, *The London Clinic Cancer Centre, 60-62 Marylebone High Street, 20-23 Devonshire Place :Summary Note on Building Materials* unpub. rep.

Museum of London, 1994 *Archaeological Site Manual 3rd edition*

Museum of London, 2002 *A research framework for London archaeology 2002*

Schofield, J, with Maloney, C, (eds), 1998 *Archaeology in the City of London 1907-1991: a guide to records of excavations by the Museum of London and its predecessors,* Archaeol Gazetteer Ser Vol 1, London

Thompson, A, Westman A, and Dyson, T (eds), 1998 *Archaeology in Greater London 1965-90: a guide to records of excavations by the Museum of London,* Archaeol Gazetteer Ser Vol 2, London

Appendix 14: An archaeological evaluation report

[DVP06]Evaluation report © MoLAS

8 NMR OASIS archaeological report form

8.1 OASIS ID: molas1-17063

Project details

Project name — London Clinic

Short description of the project — Evaluation trench in rear garden of no. 23 Devonshire Place revealed post medieval deposits containing building debris. Brick and tile fragments in this debris were dated to 16 -17th century. Natural was recorded at 24.8m OD

Project dates — Start: 10-07-2006 End: 13-07-2006

Previous/future work — Yes / Yes

Type of project — Field evaluation

Site status — Conservation Area

Site status (other) — Area of Archaeological Priority
Current Land use — Other 2 - In use as a building

Monument type — SN Post Medieval

Significant Finds — SN Post Medieval

Significant Finds — NT Post Medieval

Methods & techniques — 'Test Pits'

Development type — Urban commercial (e.g. offices, shops, banks, etc.)

Prompt — Direction from Local Planning Authority - PPG16

Position in the planning process — After full determination (eg. As a condition)

Project location

[DVP06] Evaluation Report © MoLAS

Country	England
Site location	GREATER LONDON CITY OF WESTMINSTER MARYLEBONE ST JOHNS WOOD AND MAYFAIR LONDON CLINIC
Postcode	W1
Study area	9.00 Square metres
National grid reference	TQ 52839 18204 Point
Height OD	Min: 27.60m Max: 27.60m

Project creators

Name of Organisation	MoLAS
Project originator	brief Contractor (design and execute)
Project originator	design MoLAS
Project director/manager	Ros Aitken
Project supervisor	Simon Gannon
Sponsor or funding body	London Clinic

Project archives

Physical Archive recipient	LAARC
Physical Contents	'Ceramics'
Digital Archive recipient	LAARC
Digital Contents	'Stratigraphic','Survey'
Digital Media available	'Survey','Text'
Paper Archive	LAARC

Appendix 14: An archaeological evaluation report

[DVP06] Evaluation Report © MoLAS

recipient

Paper Contents   'Stratigraphic','Survey'

Paper   Media   'Context sheet','Drawing','Map','Notebook - Excavation',' Research',' General
available   Notes','Photograph','Plan','Report','Section','Survey '

**Project
bibliography 1**

Publication type   Grey literature (unpublished document/manuscript)

Title   Evaluation at London Clinic 23 Devonshire Place

Author(s)/Editor(s)   Gannon, S.

Other bibliographic   N/A
details

Date   2006

Issuer or publisher   MoLAS

Place of issue or   N/A
publication

Description   Spiral B

Entered by   Simon Gannon (sgannon@molas.org.uk)
Entered on   4 August 2006

Please e-mail English Heritage for OASIS help and advice
© ADS 1996-2006 Created by Jo Gilham, email Last modified Friday 3 February 2006
Cite only: *http://ads.ahds.ac.uk/oasis/print.cfm* for this page

A History of The London Clinic

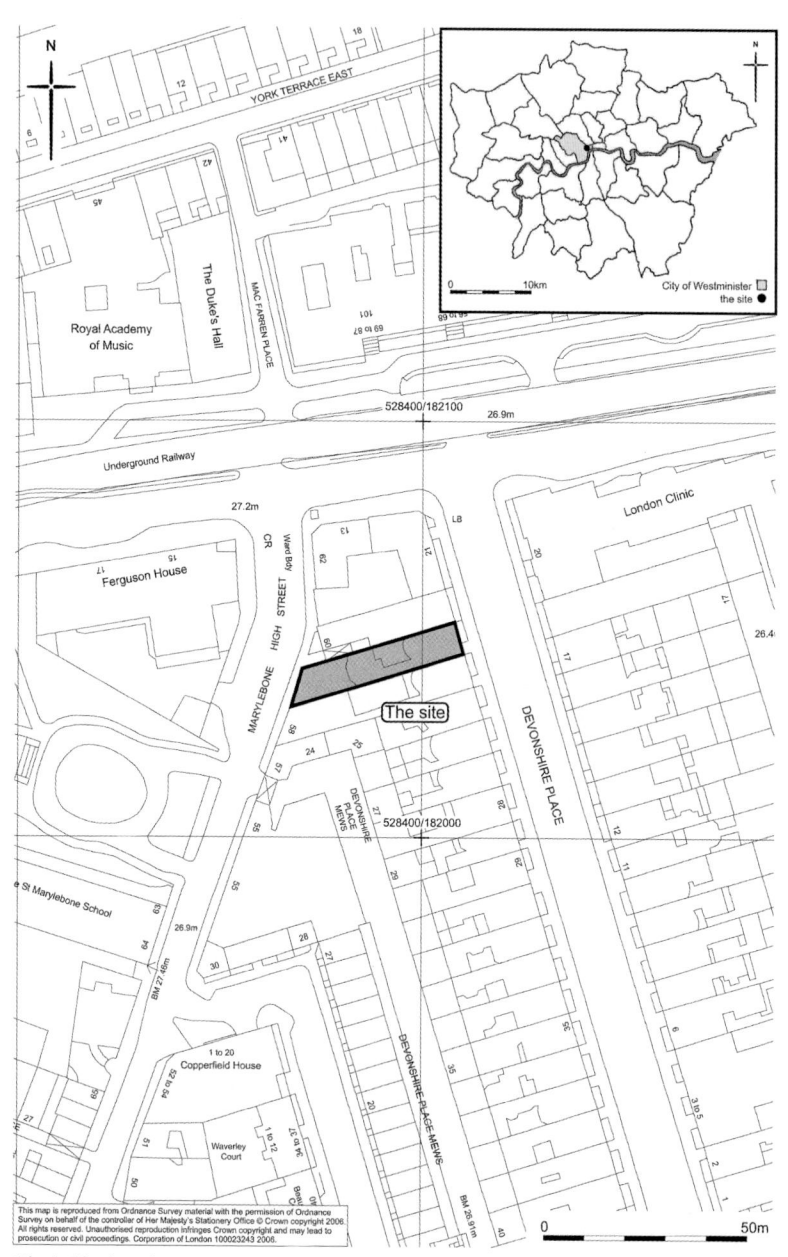

[DVP06] Evaluation Report ©MoLAS 2006

Fig 1 Site location

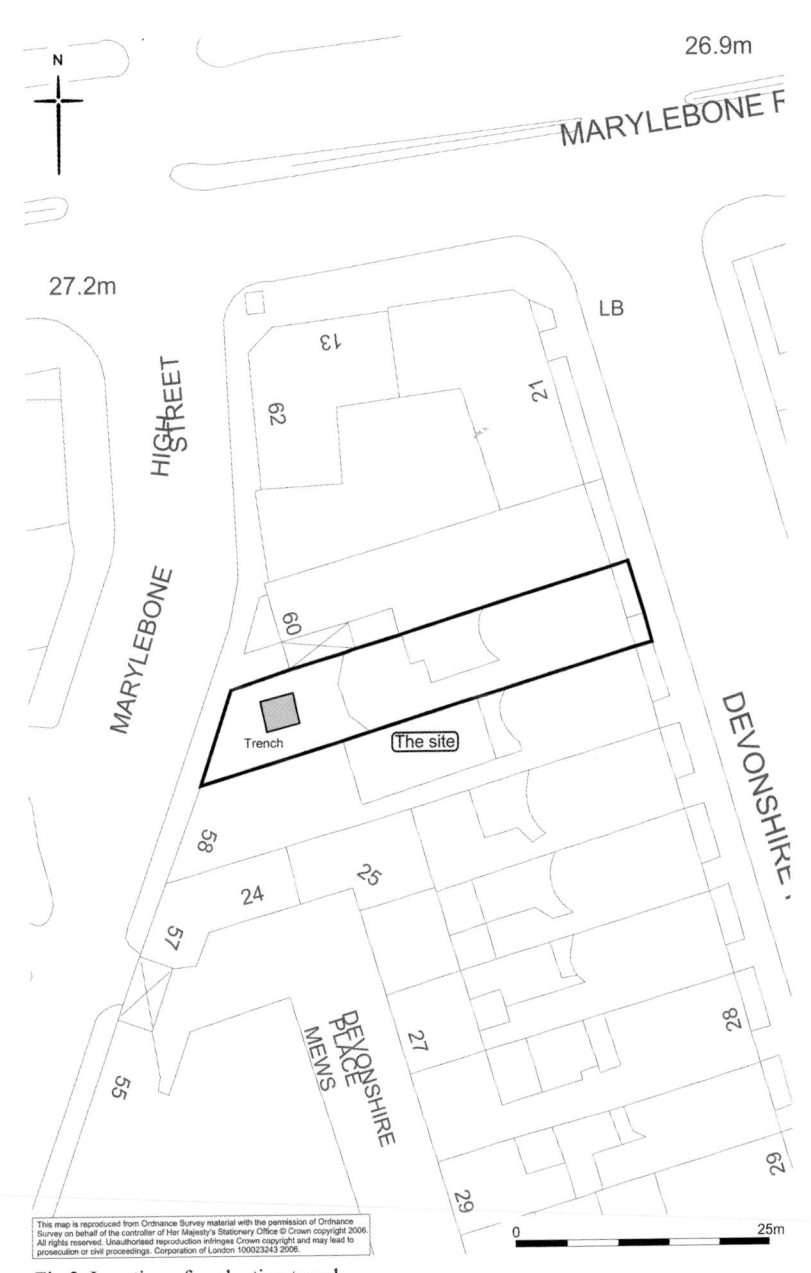

Appendix 14: An archaeological evaluation report **269**

[DVP06] Evaluation Report ©MoLAS 2006

Fig 2 Location of evaluation trench

A History of The London Clinic

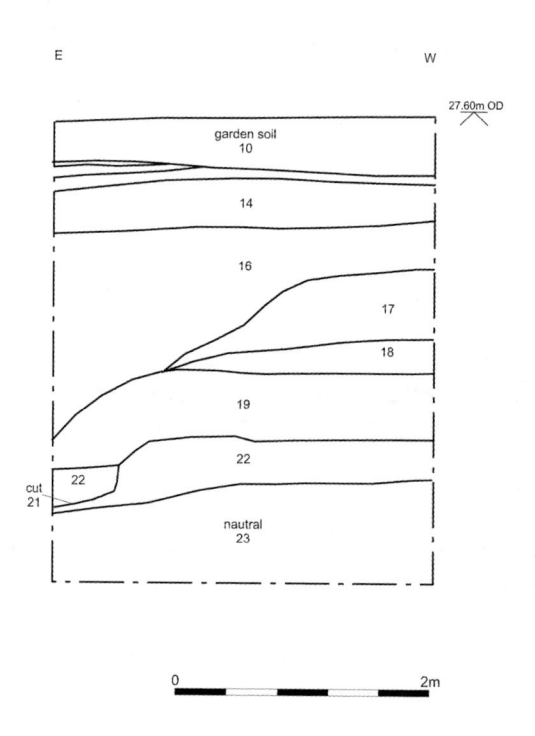

[DVP06] Evaluation Report ©MoLAS 2006

Fig 3 South facing section of evaluation trench

Reproduced with permission from the Museum of London Archaeology Service.

15

The effect of Prime Minister Anthony Eden's illness on his decision-making during the Suez crisis

Extract from *Quarterly Journal of Medicine*[1]

The effect of Prime Minister Anthony Eden's illness on his decision-making during the Suez crisis

The Right Honourable Lord Owen CH

Based on the Lord Henry Cohen History Of Medicine Lecture, University Of Liverpool, 22 February 2005

It was a misfortune not just for the Foreign Secretary, Sir Anthony Eden, but for international diplomacy, that on 12 April 1953, what should have been a routine cholecystectomy in The London Clinic, went badly wrong. The operation was undertaken on the advice of his physician, Sir Horace Evans, because of previous episodes of jaundice, abdominal pain, and the presence of gallstones. An Australian Professor, Gabriel Kune, a specialist in hepatic biliary surgery, wrote in January 2003 that Sir Horace Evans had recommended three different surgeons to Eden, all with expertise in biliary tract surgery. However, Eden chose to be operated on by the 60-year-old Mr John Basil Hume, a general surgeon at St Bartholomew's Hospital, who in Eden's words had 'removed my appendix when I was younger, and I'll go to him'.

In November 2003, an excellent review article was published by an American surgeon, Dr John Braasch, on *'Anthony Eden's (Lord Avon) Biliary Tract Saga'*. He had operated on Eden in 1970, and had had personal communication with Richard Cattell, who had undertaken the third and fourth operations on Eden in America in June 1953 and again in April 1957. Both men were associated with the Lahey Clinic in Massachusetts, and this surgical retrospection is the closest we will probably ever get to what exactly happened. Braasch very fairly quotes a minority opinion written by a retired London surgeon-knight to another US surgeon, claiming to be one of the few people who knew the facts, that while the ligature on the cystic duct had blown following the first operation (which was then evacuated in the second re-exploration operation on 29 April), Eden's 'common duct was not injured at all. When he left for America his biliary fistula had dried up, he was not jaundiced and he was perfectly well'. The letter must have been passed on to Dr Cattell. Dick Cattell was not only arguably one of the great abdominal surgeons of the 20th century, but also a gentleman, and he did not respond to the several insulting remarks contained in the letter. Another source, Sir Christopher Booth, formerly Professor of Medicine at the Royal Post Graduate Medical School, London describes Eden's first operation as a 'schoolboy howler' of surgery in which 'inadvertently [they] tied the bile duct as it comes out of the liver', resulting in the obstructive problems in the biliary tract.

According to Richard Thorpe's biography on Eden published in 2003, telling a tale that had not before been told, the surgeon, Hume, was so agitated that the operation had to be put on hold for nearly an hour to allow him to compose his nerves. After what happened in the first operation, Hume felt he could not lead the second operation, which was led by Mr Guy Blackburn, an assistant at the first. This operation has been described as 'even more tense than the first, and Eden was within a whisker of death at several stages of the lengthy and traumatic process'. The generally accepted view, supported by his official biographer, Robert Rhodes James, writing in 1986, was that Eden's biliary duct was accidentally cut and Eden was told that 'the knife slipped'.

Professor Kune further believes that there was at some stage in the London operations an injury of the right branch of the hepatic artery. This he supposes because there was found to be a high injury of the common hepatic duct in very close proximity to the right hepatic artery, and more importantly, at two re-operations in Boston, there was also a localized stricture of the right hepatic duct well away from the original duct injury site. Also, at the 1970 re-operation, the right lobe of the liver was found to be abnormally small, which suggests to Kune that at the time of the bile duct injury the right hepatic artery was also inadvertently ligated: this relative ischaemia, since the liver has a second blood supply from the portal vein, led to the development of both the stricture and the liver lobe atrophy. There is no evidence, however, that Eden's liver metabolism was affected.

Reference

The effect of Prime Minister Anthony Eden's illness on his decision-making during the Suez crisis. *QJM* 2005; **98**: 387–402.

Reproduced kind permission from Oxford University Press.

Index

Abrahams, Michael 39, 41–4, 46, 124, 170
absentee landlords 85
accommodation, residential 67
acknowledgements xv—xvi 145–6
Acts of Parliament 123
Alexandra, Princess 169
Anthony Nolan Trust 139, 141, 155
Anyan, Frank 71
appointments (office) 86, 88
Apps, Paul 120, 131
archaeological evaluation report 245–70
architect (CH Biddulph Pinchard) 18–19
Atholl, eighth duke 25–7
Auden, WH, qq 5–6
automobiles 93–4
Avery Jones, Francis 124
Avery Jones, John 124

Bader, Douglas 93–4
Barker, Andrew 124
Beecroft, Tony 44
Belloc, Hilaire, *quoted* 8–9
boards, governors and trustees 45, 151–2
Boden, Betty (matron) 65–9
Bridgland, Aynsley 26–8
    obituary 181–4
Bristow, Aubrey 106
Buckley, Hoda 72
buildings 17–24
    Cancer Centre, computer images 48–9
    Devonshire Place façade 20
    Devonshire Street frontage 18
    dining rooms 74–6, 86
    ground floor plan 23
    Harley Street, Northern end 18
    housekeeping 80
    maintenance 81
    Marylebone Road frontage 17
    operating theatres 22, 92, 99–108
    proposed 1963 development 23–4
    purchasing and stores 81–2
    refurbishment and development 38
    stone carvings 20, 21
Bull, James 110
Bullivant, Karen 44
Burgess, Brian 124

Cancer Centre, computer images 48–9
capital equipment 81–2
catering 73–8
Cavendish family 2
Cavendish Harley Estate 6
celebrities 55–60
    openings of departments 165–70
    royal patients 55–7
    royalty 165–6, 169
    sports 60, 167
    stage, screen and radio stars 58–9, 167–9

chairmen 149
   Medical Advisory Committee 154
Chalstrey, John (Lord Mayor of London) 113, 115, 167
charitable donations and support 141
charitable status 27, 147–8, 155–8
Charles (Prince of Wales) 165
Chief Executive 44, 123–4, 149
children's services 51
Churchill, Winston 62
clinical specialities, current 140, 141
committee structure of LC 159–60
computed tomography 112
Connaught, Arthur (Prince) 55
construction costs, London Clinic 12
consultants
   numbers 142
   past 91
consulting rooms
   licences 12, 85
   No. 149 Harley Street 83
current clinical/diagnostic specialities 140, 141

Dawson, Lord, of Penn 95, 97
day care 139
Dettori, Frankie 60, 167
development and future plans for LC 137–42
Devonshire, Duchess of 137, 166, 169–70
Devonshire family 2, 137, 166, 169–70
Devonshire Place
   1793 xii
   consulting rooms 47–8, 133, 137
Devonshire Street
   1793 and 2007 4
   west frontage 18
dining rooms 74–6, 86
dogs 94–5
Douglas, Lewis (US Ambassador) 60
Dove Cottage 49
Drury, Ian 167
Dunhill, Thomas 93
Dutton, Sylvia (matron) 65–6

Eden, Anthony (Prime Minister) 57
   illness, and Suez decision-making 58, 271–2

Eisenhower, Dwight D 128
Elizabeth II 56
Elizabeth (Queen Mother) viii, 88
endoscopy 113–16
Executive Board 152
   formation 43–5
explosive ordnance, threat assessment 185–244

fees 12
Florence Nightingale Hospital 5
Francis-Saati, Pierre Maher 72
future plans for LC 137–42

George, Patricia 71
George V 12
Getty, Paul 35–7, 95
Getty, Victoria 166
Gibbs, Christopher 35–6
Gillies, Harold 100, 129
Gilmour, Ian 40
Gloucester, Duchess of 170
Goldstone, John 106
Gorecki, Wanda 114, 115
governors and trustees 45, 151–2
Grantham, VA (Chairman 1966–68) 28, 29
Griffiths, John 91, 93, 118, 129

Hallowes, Odette 128
Hallums, Amanda (matron) 44, 68–9
Harley House, endoscopy unit 113
Harley, Robert 3–4
Harley Street 5–6
   in 1928 8
   bomb damage 127
   development (1753 on) 5–6
   new additions to LC 137
   No. 114–120 89–90
   No. 119 89
   No. 149 (consultants' offices) 83, 89, 134
   No. 149 future plans 137
   Northern end 18
Hathorn, Jean 127
Henderson, Laura (matron) 65–6, 69
Hepworth, Barbara (sculptor) 101–2
Hickinbotham, Tom (Chairman 1968–78) 28, 29, 117

Index

high dependency unit 106–7
Hill, Tony Fenton 113
history of LC 1–10
Hoare, Reginald 95
Horder, Lord, of Ashford 95–7
hospitals, specialist 11
house governors 123–4, 149
Howard de Walden Estate 5–6
    suggested purchase of LC from Trustees 36
Hunterian Society collection 89
Husband, Janet 112
hydrotherapy unit 36

imaging 112
information technology 125–6
intensive therapy unit 36, 106–7
interpreters 72
Irvine, Gillian 44

Jacomb, Jean (matron) 64–5
James, D Geraint 89
Jenner, Michael 32–3, 38, 106, 123

Kaldos, Rania 72
Kent, Richard (Dick) 37, 123
Kings Fund certification (private sector) 38, 46
Kirby, Roger 105
kitchens 73–7
Knox, Thomas Daniel (Lord Ranfurly, sixth earl) 31–2

lease, London Clinic 12, 25
Lewis, Joan (matron) 56, 61–2, 65
licences 12, 85
logos, old and new 50
London Clinic, *see also* buildings
London Clinic Cancer Centre, computer images 48–9
London Clinic Medical Journal, The 129–32
    listings of clinical articles 171–8
    listings of non-clinical articles 179–80

MacFeat, W Ogilvie 110, 114
McGill, Ivan 99
McIndoe, Archibald Hector 100
magnetic resonance imaging 112

Maingot, Rodney 129–30
Makins twins 15
Margaret, HRH Princess 112, 166
Mary, Queen 12
Marylebone 1–3
    bomb damage 128
Marylebone Estate, map (1708) 5
maternity services 51
matrons 61–2, 67, 149–50
    office 68–9
Medical Advisory Committee (MAC) 39
    chairmen 154
    members 2007 153
Medsafe 125
Menderes, Adnam (Prime Minister of Turkey) 129
Miller, Malcolm 42–4, 123, 125, 170
minimally invasive theatre unit 108
mission and philosophy 147–8
Morgan, Clifford Naunton 105
Morris, Ernest 123
Morson, Basil 65
Moynihan, Lord 14
Muir, Edward 106

newsletters 131
nurse education, and St Bartholomew's 67
nursing 61–70
    accomodation 62–5
    education 67–8
    uniforms 62–4
nursing homes, private 12

opening ceremony 12
openings of departments 165–70
operating theatres 22, 92, 99–108
Operations Board 151, 151–2
organizational charts, London Clinic 161

Parkes, Alan 106
pathology 117–20
patients
    and charitable status of LC 27, 147–8, 155–8
    free treatment 157
    numbers 141–2, 156
    requirement(s) of patients 11–12, 52–4

Patil, Krishna 105
Perkins, Kathy 124–5, 131
pharmacy 120–2
phlebotomy 72
physiotherapy 71–2
Piggott, Lester 60
Pinchard, CHB (architect) 18–19
Pinochet, Augusto (President of Chile), at LC 87
porters 79
Portland Estate
   Howard de Walden Estate 5–6
   origins 4
private nursing homes 12
professional life 6–9
progressive care unit 106–7
purchasing and stores 81–2
purpose/philosophy of LC 45

radiology, radiotherapy 109–11
Ramsden, James (Chairman) 33–5, 37–9
Ranfurly, sixth earl (TD Knox) 31–2
receivership 25–7
receptionists 79–80
residential accommodation 67
restaurant 75
Roberts, Mike 44, 126
Ross, Harvey 93, 105
Ross, James Paterson 93–4
royal celebrities 165–6, 169
royal patients 55–7, 88

St Bartholomew's Hospital, nurse education scheme 67
Scharlieb, Mary Ann Dacomb 84
Seear, Tiba 112

Second World War 127–31
Shah, Sanjay 44
Shingles, Rene 134
Sims, Mike (purchasing and stores) 81–2
Sinclair, Archie 128
Slevin, Maurice 138
snake sculpture 36
specialty user groups (2007) 154
sports celebrities 60, 167
stage, screen and radio stars 58–9
Suez crisis 129
   decision-making (Anthony Eden, Prime Minister) 58, 271–2
switchboard 79–80

Taylor, Elizabeth 59
Terrace restaurant 75
Todd, Ian 106
trustees and governors 45, 151–2
Turner, Sian 134
Tyburn, Manor 1–2

Ulster Terrace offices 47–8

Waite, Ron 125
Warner, Helen 110
Weizman, Chaim and Vera 58
Williams, Roger 139
Wimpole Street (1793) xii
Windsor, Duke and Duchess 56
Winslet, Marc 139
Wood, Paul 38
Worthington, Mike 125
Wright, Dickson 59, 127

York, Duke and Duchess 12–13